# The First-Time Mom's Blueprint:

*Pregnancy Guide for First Time Moms & The Postpartum Handbook*

*(2 Manuscripts in 1)*

**MOMMY'S ANGELS**
EDITORIAL STAFF
GROW YOUR TODDLER TO THE BEST!

## ABOUT MOMMY'S ANGELS

### GROW YOUR TODDLER TO THE BEST

Are you a first-time mother? Or are you planning for the arrival of your baby? Well, you are not alone on this exciting journey of your life. Of course, we understand that this period can be full of doubts and questions, which is why **MOMMY'S ANGELS** is a must-read for every young mother.

While you will have people around you who would want to help you, the surest way to understand what happens with your body, emotions, baby's health and everything related to pregnancy and even postpartum, is having a reliable personal guide by you 24/7 all-through the pregnancy period – whenever the need arises.

Although you are the only that will know how you are feeling or what you inside you, the thought of having to filter through the countless books on pregnancy and parenting can sometimes be very daunting – especially during these forty weeks, the period of breastfeeding as well as the first few months of your baby. The **MOMMY'S ANGELS Series** include a vast range of book collections and vital tips that you need to help you grow your toddler to the best.

While these books are not intended to be a mandatory regime that you must follow, the comments, stories, and experiences of pediatricians, psychologists, gynecologists and other mothers like you, will help you enjoy the best adventure of your life.

Visit our various sections to find the best pregnancy books, including those for your toddlers and young children! You will undoubtedly find the books very relevant and interesting, too!

Learn the most effective ways to grow your toddler with **MOMMY'S ANGELS Book Collections.**

## MOMMY'S ANGELS
EDITORIAL STAFF
GROW YOUR TODDLER TO THE BEST!

© Copyright 2020 by Mommy's Angels - All rights reserved.

The content contained within this book may not be reproduced, duplicated, or transmitted without direct written permission from the author or the publisher.

Under no circumstances will any blame or legal responsibility be held against the publisher, or author, for any damages, reparation, or monetary loss due to the information contained within this book. Either directly or indirectly. You are responsible for your own choices, actions, and results.

Legal Notice:

This book is copyright protected. This book is only for personal use. You cannot amend, distribute, sell, use, quote or paraphrase any part, or the content within this book, without the consent of the author or publisher.

Disclaimer Notice:

Please note the information contained within this document is for educational and entertainment purposes only. All effort has been executed to present accurate, up to date, and reliable, complete information. No warranties of any kind are declared or implied. Readers acknowledge that the author is not engaging in the rendering of legal, financial, medical, or professional advice. The content within this book has been derived from various sources. Please consult a licensed professional before attempting any techniques outlined in this book.

By reading this document, the reader agrees that under no circumstances is the author responsible for any losses, direct or indirect, which are incurred as a result of the use of the information contained within this document, including, but not limited to, — errors, omissions, or inaccuracies.

# Table of Contents

## Pregnancy Guide for First Time Moms

**Preface of the Book** ................................................................... 19

**Chapter 1: The Journey Of Maternity** ........................................ 20

  The Visit to The Doctor ............................................................ 21

    Understanding Your Medical History ..................................... 21

    Evaluating Your Mental And Physical Health ......................... 22

  Some Commonly Asked Questions Regarding Pregnancy ............. 24

    How to achieve ideal body weight ........................................ 24

    Revising Your Medications ................................................... 25

    Using Nutritional Supplements ............................................. 28

    Understanding The Need For Vaccination And Immunity ........ 28

    Stop Using Birth Control Methods ........................................ 29

    When To Worry About Infertility .......................................... 30

  Timing Is Everything In Reproduction ........................................ 31

    Locating Ovulation .............................................................. 32

  Always Use an Effective Approach ............................................ 34

**Chapter 2:** ................................................................................ 36

**Hurray! You Think You Are Pregnant** ........................................ 36

  The Right Signs of Pregnancy ................................................... 36

  Determining If You Are Pregnant ............................................... 38

    Do-it-yourself Test for Answers ............................................ 39

    Visiting the Doctor for Answers ............................................ 39

  Finding the Right Doctor .......................................................... 40

    Understand Different Options ............................................... 40

  Right Questions to Ask Before You Make A Decision .................. 42

    Finding Your Due Date ........................................................ 43

  Some Old Pregnancy Myths That You Need to Know .................. 44

## Chapter 3: Prepare Yourself for Pregnancy ............... 48
### Plan Parental Visit ............... 49
### Prepare Yourself for Emotional Changes ............... 51
#### Increased Mood Swings ............... 51
#### Prepare for Leg Cramps ............... 52
#### Vaginal discharge ............... 53
#### Increased Backaches ............... 53
#### Coping with Stress ............... 54
### How Medications, Drugs, And Alcohol Affect Your Body ............... 54
#### Medications: ............... 55
#### Smoking ............... 56
#### Drinking liquor ............... 57
#### Utilizing recreational/unlawful medications ............... 58
### Making Lifestyle Changes ............... 59
#### Spoiling yourself with excellence medicines ............... 59
#### Using Steam Rooms, Saunas and Hot Tubs While Pregnant ............... 62
#### Voyaging ............... 63
#### Getting dental consideration ............... 65
#### Engaging in Sexual Relations ............... 67
### Working When You Are Pregnant ............... 68
#### Thinking about work-related risks ............... 69
#### Getting pregnant and the law ............... 71

## Chapter 4: Exercise and Dietary Requirements for A Pregnant Woman ............... 73
### Healthy Weight Gain ............... 74
#### Understanding How Much Weight Is Good ............... 74
#### Knowing your infant's weight gain ............... 75
### Understanding What You Are Eating ............... 77
#### Utilizing the USDA Food Guide Pyramid ............... 77
#### Enhancing your eating diet ............... 81
#### Is caffeine safe during pregnancy? ............... 82
### Knowing Which Food Items Are Safe ............... 85

    Some harmful nourishments to look out for ........................... 85
    Popular Food Myths to Know About ......................................... 86
    Considering Special Dietary Needs ......................................... 89
    Eating right, veggie lover style .................................................. 89
    Fighting Constipation ................................................................. 90
    Managing diabetes ..................................................................... 90
  Adjusting to Your Body's Progressions ........................................... 91
    Excersing Without Trying Too Hard ......................................... 93
    Diverse pregnant women exercises ......................................... 95

## Chapter 5: The First Trimester ...................................... 97

  A New Life Begins ............................................................................ 98
  Know that body changes you should expect in pregnancy ............... 98
    Changes in the Breast................................................................. 99
    Fatigue....................................................................................... 100
    Sickness During the Day ......................................................... 100
    Bloating..................................................................................... 100
    Urination Issues........................................................................ 101
    Headaches ................................................................................ 101
    Constipation ............................................................................. 102
  The First Prenatal Appointment ..................................................... 102
    Lifestyle .................................................................................... 103
    The last menstrual period ....................................................... 103
    Gynecological History ............................................................. 103
    Infertility treatment................................................................. 104
    Medical Problems .................................................................... 104
    Family Medical History ........................................................... 104
    Ethnic roots .............................................................................. 105
    Screening for cystic fibrosis .................................................... 106
    Thinking about the physical test ............................................ 107
    Looking at the standard tests ................................................. 107
    Prepare for the prick: Blood tests .......................................... 107

Ultrasound in the first trimester ............................................. 109
   Coming up next are assessed during a first-trimester ultrasound test: ........................................................................... 110
Perceiving Causes for Concern ............................................... 111
   Bleeding ........................................................................ 111
   Miscarriage .................................................................... 113
   Ectopic pregnancy ......................................................... 114

## Chapter 6: The Second Trimester ............................................ 116

Finding How Your Baby Is Developing ..................................... 117
   Dressing in maternity clothing ....................................... 119
Understanding Your Changing Body ........................................ 121
   Distraction and awkwardness ........................................ 121
   Gas ................................................................................ 122
   Hair and nail development ............................................. 122
   Acid reflux .................................................................... 123
   Lower stomach/crotch torment ..................................... 124
   Nasal clog ..................................................................... 124
   Nosebleeds and bleeding gums ..................................... 125
   Skin changes ................................................................ 125
   Checking In: Prenatal Visits ........................................... 126
Perceiving Causes for Concern in the second trimester ............ 127
   Bleeding ........................................................................ 127
   Fetal variation from the norm ....................................... 128
   Inept cervix ................................................................... 128
   When you need to start looking for help! ...................... 130
For Dads: Watching Mom Grow ............................................... 130

## Chapter 7: The Last Three Months of Pregnancy .................... 133

Your Baby Gets Ready for Birth ............................................... 134
   Movin' and shakin': Fetal developments ........................ 135
   Utilizing the breathing muscles .................................... 136
   Hiccupping in utero ...................................................... 137
Staying aware of Your Changing Body ..................................... 137

- Accidents ..................................................................................... 138
- Braxton-Hicks ............................................................................. 138
- A pregnant lady knows no outsiders ...................................... 139
- Carpal passage disorder ........................................................... 140
- Weakness ..................................................................................... 140
- Hemorrhoids ............................................................................... 141
- Insomnia ...................................................................................... 142
- Feeling the infant "drop" ......................................................... 143
- Pregnancy rashes and tingles ................................................. 145
- How to Plan for breastfeeding ............................................... 146
- Sciatica ......................................................................................... 148
- Brevity of breath ........................................................................ 148
- Tackling Stretch imprints ......................................................... 149
- Planning for Labor .................................................................... 149

Making labor preparation ............................................................. 151
- Requesting a C-Section ............................................................ 151

Perceiving Causes for Concern .................................................... 152
- Bleeding ....................................................................................... 153
- Breech introduction .................................................................. 153
- Diminished amniotic liquid volume ...................................... 154
- Fetal development issues ........................................................ 155
- Releasing amniotic liquid ........................................................ 156
- Preeclampsia .............................................................................. 157
- Understanding Preterm work ................................................. 157

## Chapter 8: What to expect from Labor process ............... 159

How to know if Labor is real or not! ......................................... 160
- Seeing changes before labor starts ....................................... 160
- What is real and fake labor ..................................................... 162

Understanding when you need to see the doctor .................. 163
- Checking for work with an inner test ................................... 164

The main characteristics of Labor .............................................. 164

 First stage ............................................................................... 168

 Potential issues during labor's first stage ................................. 168

## Chapter 9: Bringing The Baby In the World .......................... 170

 Understanding the Vaginal Delivery ........................................... 171

  Pushing the baby ................................................................... 172

  Getting an episiotomy ........................................................... 174

 Taking care of delayed second-arrange labor ........................... 175

 The defining moment: Delivering your infant ............................ 175

  Delivering the placenta ......................................................... 176

  Fixing your perineum ............................................................ 176

  Helping Nature: Operative Vaginal Delivery .......................... 177

 Understanding Cesarean Delivery ............................................. 178

  Getting anesthesia ................................................................ 180

  Taking a gander at purposes behind cesarean delivery ............. 180

  Congrats! You Did It! ............................................................ 183

  Shaking after delivery ........................................................... 184

  Know more about postpartum bleeding ................................ 184

 Checking In: Baby's First Doctor Visit ....................................... 186

## Chapter 10: Dealing with Special Concerns ......................... 189

 How Age matters in pregnancy .................................................. 189

  Becoming pregnant in age 30 or over .................................... 190

 Having Multiple Babies ............................................................... 192

 Differentiating multiples as identical or fraternal ....................... 194

 Precautions at the time of labor and delivery ............................. 200

 How to tackle premature birth of twins ...................................... 205

 Planning another baby ................................................................ 207

  Differentiating between each pregnancy .............................. 207

  Giving birth after C-section ................................................... 209

  Belonging from a Non-traditional Family ............................... 211

 How to prepare your children for newborn ................................ 212

  Explaining Pregnancy ............................................................ 212

    Arrangement for babysitting during delivery ............................ 213

# Chapter 11: Breastfeeding .................................................... 215

  Breast-Feeding and its Importance .......................................... 217
    The process of milk production ............................................... 217
  Benefits for Mother ................................................................. 218
    Delay in Periods ...................................................................... 218
    Helps in faster recovery ......................................................... 218
    Long-term Health Benefits ..................................................... 219
    Benefits for Baby ................................................................... 219
    Protection against disease ...................................................... 219
    Complete Nutrition ................................................................ 220
    Protects a child from obesity .................................................. 220
    Easy to digest ......................................................................... 220
    Other major benefits ............................................................. 220
  Major Pros and Cons of Breast-feeding ..................................... 221
  Situations when breast-feeding is not possible .......................... 223
    Vitamin D requirement .......................................................... 224
    Tips for your convenience ...................................................... 225
    Take advice when you require ............................................... 225
    Additional supplies required .................................................. 226
    Don't feel panic ..................................................................... 226
    Always breast-feed your baby in a comfortable position ............ 227
    Baby feeding positions .......................................................... 227
    Breast-feeding to multiple babies ........................................... 229
    Basics of Nursing ................................................................... 230
  Maintain your Health ............................................................... 232
  Tips for Breast Care ................................................................. 233
    Other Methods of Pumping Your Breasts: ................................ 236
    How regularly will you utilize the breast pump? ...................... 236
    How quickly you need to pump? ............................................ 237
    How much does a breast pump cost? ..................................... 237

- Is it easy to assemble and ship the breast pump? ..................... 237
- How can I adjust the suction? ............................................... 238
- What is the correct size of the breast shields? ......................... 238
- How to Store Breast Milk .................................................... 238
- To store breast milk, what kind of container is required? ........... 238
- What's the ideal approach to store expressed bosom milk? ........ 239
- Can I mix freshly expressed breast milk with stored milk? ......... 239
- For how many days can I keep expressed milk? ...................... 239
- How would I defrost frozen breast milk? ................................. 240
- Is there anything else to know about breast milk storage? ......... 241
- Continuing your routine work ............................................... 241
- Bottle-feeding ................................................................... 241
- Advantages and Disadvantages of Bottle-feeding ..................... 242
  - How to start bottle-feeding: ............................................... 245
  - Preparing formula milk: .................................................... 246
  - Get into right position: ..................................................... 248

## Chapter 12: Ten Important Points About Pregnancy ............... 250

- Pregnancy Lasts Longer than Nine Months ............................. 250
- Others Can Drive You Crazy ................................................ 251
- You Feel Exhausted in the First Trimester .............................. 251
- Round Ligament Pain Really Hurts ........................................ 252
- Your Belly Becomes a Hand Magnet ...................................... 252
- Hemorrhoids Are a Royal Pain in the Butt ............................... 253
- Now and then Women Poop While Pushing ............................. 253
- The Weight Stays On after the Baby Comes Out ...................... 253
- Medical clinic Pads are Relics from Your Mother's Era ................ 253
- Breast Engorgement Really Sucks and Breast-encouraging Can Be a Production ....................................................................... 254

## Conclusion: ........................................................................ 255

# The Postpartum Handbook

**Chapter 1: Postpartum Introduction ............................................. 259**
- Physical Changes ............................................................ 260
  - Breasts and Lactation ................................................. 260
  - Change to the Uterus .................................................. 261
  - Vagina, Cervix, and Perineum ......................................... 261
  - Immune Response ....................................................... 262
  - Pain Control .......................................................... 262
  - Changes in Nutrition .................................................. 263
  - Changes due to C-section .............................................. 264
- Emotional Changes .......................................................... 265

**Chapter 2: Types of Postpartum ................................................ 266**
- Postpartum Blues ........................................................... 266
  - Cause of postpartum blues ............................................. 267
- Postpartum Depression ...................................................... 269
- Postpartum Anxiety ......................................................... 276
  - Causes of Postpartum Anxiety .......................................... 277
- Postpartum Obsessive-Compulsive Disorder (OCD) ............................. 279
  - Causes of Postpartum OCD .............................................. 279
- Postpartum Bipolar Disorder ................................................ 281
  - Causes of Bipolar Disorder ............................................ 281
- Postpartum Panic Disorder .................................................. 283
  - Causes of Postpartum Panic Disorder ................................... 284
- Postpartum Psychosis ....................................................... 286
  - Causes of Postpartum Psychosis ........................................ 287
- Postpartum Post-Traumatic Stress Disorder .................................. 288

**Chapter 3: How to Overcome Negative Thoughts .................................. 290**
- Understanding Your Concerns and Releasing Negative Thoughts ................ 298
- Tips to overcome negative thoughts at home ................................. 301

**Chapter 4: Doctor's Help ...................................................... 306**

- Pharmacological treatment ................................................................. 306
  - Antidepressants .......................................................... 306
- Breastfeeding Considerations ................................................ 309
- Non-Pharmacological Treatment ............................................ 310
  - Interpersonal Psychotherapy ................................... 311
  - Cognitive-Behavioral Therapy ................................ 312
  - Dialectical Behavioral Therapy ............................... 312
  - How you should talk to your doctor about postpartum ............. 315

## Chapter 5: Postpartum in Fathers .................................................. 318
- Fathers' Experience After Birth ............................................. 319
- Hormonal Changes in Fathers ................................................ 320
- Neural and Behavioral Changes in Fathers .............................. 320
- Symptoms of Postpartum in Fathers ...................................... 321
- Effects of Postpartum Depression in Fathers .......................... 323
- Video Feedback Interventions ................................................ 324
- Screening for Father's Postpartum ......................................... 326

## Chapter 6: Problems Faced in Postpartum and Their Solutions 329
- Problems in Postpartum ......................................................... 329
- Emotional changes ................................................................. 330
- Physical Changes .................................................................... 336

## Chapter 7: Vaginal Discharge ........................................................ 342
- Weight problems .................................................................... 342
  - Constipation ............................................................. 343
  - Pelvic floor and bladder problems ........................... 343
- Pain in the perineal area ....................................................... 345
- Change in body size ............................................................... 346

## Chapter 8: Preventive Measures for Postpartum ....................... 349
- Meditation .............................................................................. 349
- Placenta Therapy ................................................................... 350
- Acupuncture and acupressure ............................................... 352
- Prenatal Vitamins .................................................................. 354

Share your feelings ............................................................... 361
## Chapter 9: Effects of Postpartum on Newborns ...................... 363
Infant Development and Mother's Depression ............................ 363
   Mother/newborn communication ............................................. 363
   Psychological improvement .................................................... 364
Maternal depression and developmental outcome of toddlers and preschoolers ................................................................................. 364
   Conduct advancement ........................................................ 364
   Intellectual advancement .................................................... 365
Maternal depression and developmental outcome of school-age children .......................................................................................... 365
   Social advancement ............................................................ 366
   Family treatment ................................................................. 368
## Chapter 10: Advantage of Partner Support in Postpartum ...... 369
Accomplice Support ................................................................... 369
Grown-up Romantic Attachment Patterns ................................. 373
## Conclusion: ................................................................................ 380

# Pregnancy Guide for First Time Moms

*Your Know-It-All Guide For The Next Nine Months And Beyond*

**MOMMY'S ANGELS**
EDITORIAL STAFF
GROW YOUR TODDLER TO THE BEST!

# Preface of the Book

Do you remember the time you started driving? The time you got married? These events are of utter importance in anyone's life. Among all the events in anyone's life – nothing can beat the joy of childbirth. You will feel happy that you are bringing a new person to this world and have endured nine months' long struggle to ensure that the baby is healthy. You will go to the world's end to make sure that the newborn is healthy and you will protect him or her at any cost, to have a wonderful beginning, and to have unbreakable bond with your baby.

This book is designed to give the scientifically correct knowledge to first-time parents and make sure that we provide adequate knowledge regarding this memorable experience in their life. This book is easy to comprehend, and all the data is formatted in such a way that the readers can get substantial information about the process of making babies.

This book is geared towards the woman who is considering pregnancy or already pregnant and needs more information about the process. This book will also be helpful for the partner of the mother-to-be, and you may also read this book if you love someone who is pregnant. If you fall into these criteria, the nine months' pregnancy journey is the right book for you.

# Chapter 1:
# The Journey Of Maternity

*You will learn:*

---

*Evaluate Your Health And Family Past*

*Preparing The Body For Maternity*

*Get Knowledge Of The Vaccines And Medications*

---

If you are pregnant, you are going to start a wonderful and exciting adventure of your life. If you are planning to get pregnant, you will be a little nervous about the next nine months, but this guide will help you to prepare for this extraordinary journey.

This chapter will focus on all the details that you need to know before you conceive. We will highlight the vaccines and medications that you will need to know if you are pregnant. The first step of getting pregnant is to visit your medical practitioner and discuss your health and family history. In this way, you will know whether you are ready for pregnancy or if you need to lose weight, avoid using some medication or you need to quit smoking. Some medications can be harmful to the female body when they are pregnant or breastfeeding. We will provide some elementary advice regarding the best way to conceive and will also help you understand the concept of infertility.

# The Visit to The Doctor

The embryo will go through different changes since the time you miss your period and know that you are pregnant. You need to know that the brain and heart have already been developed in the first two or three weeks. Your overall health plays a vital factor in the development of these organs, and being healthy before you conceive will surely help the newborn in the early stages of development. The initial or preconception visit is to make sure that you are ready for the pregnancy journey, and your body is tuned up to hold a baby. You can schedule this visit during a routine visit of the gynecologist. During the yearly visit to the doctor, remember to tell the doctor that you are planning to have a baby. If the annual test is due for a long time, make an appointment with the doctor. It is advised that both parents should visit the doctor so that the medical histories of both parents can be discussed. Do not worry if you have not done a preconception visit and are pregnant; you can discuss all these topics in your first prenatal visit.

**Understanding Your Medical History**
When you visit the doctor for the preconception visit, the doctor will analyze your medical history and also make sure that you and your baby are ready for the pregnancy. The doctor is likely to ask you about the following things:

**Asking about your ethic routes:** There might be some problems with certain populations. In the preconception visit, the doctor will ask about the medical history of your grandparents and parents. This is a common question to ask when you are planning to have a child. There are certain advantages of discussing the ancestral history and by this, you and your partner will be saved from pregnancy-related issues before you conceive.

**Your Family History:** learning about the family history will inform the doctor about any complication that you might get once you are pregnant. Diseases such as diabetes and spina bifida run in the family, and these can complicate your pregnancy. When the baby is developing in your body, your doctor will know which medicine to give you based on your family history.

**Gynecologic History and Previous Pregnancies:** Discussing your previous pregnancies will help your doctor to prepare you for the future. The doctor will ask you about your previous single and multiple pregnancies and will also inquire about any miscarriage that you had in the past. The doctor will know about the previous problems that you faced in the past, such as high blood pressure and vaginal bleeding and this will help them guide you in a better way regarding your pregnancy journey.

**Evaluating Your Mental And Physical Health**

Many women who are planning to become mothers do not have any complications and their bodies are fit to hold a baby. However, the preconception visits help the doctor to plan your pregnancy journey and make sure that you have an uncomplicated and healthy pregnancy. When the doctor evaluates your body, he/she will let you know about the ideal weight for a pregnant woman, the multivitamins that you should take and how to exercise properly to ensure a healthy child.

## PELVIC EXAM

Some women suffer from medical problems that can affect their pregnancy and the medical practitioner will ask you about the medicines that you take to ensure that your body is ready for birth. The doctor will ask you whether you suffer from high blood pressure, diabetes and increased fatigue. These things can complicate pregnancy. If you suffer from high blood pressure, then the doctor will make sure that they change your medication before you are pregnant. Controlling blood pressure is not an easy job and may require changing medication multiple times. Other problems, such as epilepsy, need to be controlled before you start your pregnancy journey. The doctor will advise you to become pregnant when you have fewer symptoms of these diseases.

When you get to the doctor for the first checkup, the doctor will ask if you smoke, drink or use any recreational drug. You should not feel that the doctor is interrogating you; this is just some precautionary questions that help the doctor to evaluate your physical and mental health. With this knowledge, the doctor will give you the best tips to drop these habits to ensure a safe pregnancy. They will advise some support groups or medications that can help you quit these habits. Apart from this, it is also advised that you discuss the over the counter drugs that you use and also share your dietary habits with the doctor. The physician will recommend a PAP smear test during the visit.

## Some Commonly Asked Questions Regarding Pregnancy

The preconception visit is the time when you will have a lot of questions in your mind regarding pregnancy and this is the best time when you can clear all your confusion about pregnancy. In this section, we will focus on all the commonly asked questions – these questions are related to the tablets, child control medications, vaccination, and body weight.

### How to achieve ideal body weight

Women are always concerned about their body mass when they are planning to conceive. well, this is an important factor that you need to consider. Pregnancy will go smooth for women who are not too thin or too fat. The underweight women have the risk of giving birth to low birth weight babies and the women who are fat may risk of having high blood pressure or developing diabetes during their pregnancy. Such conditions can lead to birth via cesarean section. You need to make sure that you reach a normal weight before you are pregnant. You should not try to lose weight after you have got pregnant as this can affect the child's health. On the other hand, adding pounds when you are pregnant is fairly difficult as well.

**Revising Your Medications**

There are many medications that are safe to take when you are pregnant. When you are taking medication which is essential for your health and well-being – discuss them with your medical practitioner. You need to have a discussion with the doctor before you stop using these medications. So, it is essential that you discuss all the medications that you are using and the doctor will change the medication if it is putting a lot of risk for your baby or your health during pregnancy. The medications that are considered safe during the pregnancy include:

- Aspirin
- Antiemetic
- Minor antidepressants
- Zidovudine
- Acetaminophen
- Antihistamines
- Acyclovir
- Penicillin

Some medications that general women are confused about are listed below:

**Ibuprofen:** You will be relaxed to know that mild use of Motrin and Advil are considered safe during the pregnancy and does not affect newborn. Although these medicines may be safe for short term use, you need to make sure that you **avoid chronic use** of these medications, especially in the last months of the pregnancy. These medicines tends to affect the blood circulation and platelet function in the body and put a strain on the kidney function. As the baby's kidney works the same as your kidneys, so avoid using them in large quantities.

**Bupropion:** Bupropion is a medication that is used to quit smoking and some people also used it as an antidepressant. There is very little research on the effects of this medication during pregnancy but the available data shows that there is no harmful effect of using this medicine during pregnancy. This medicine **should not** be used as an antidepressant during pregnancy.

**Tetracycline:** This medicine should be **avoided** during the last months of pregnancy; this medicine may cause the newborn baby's teeth to turn yellow.

**Antidepressants:** There is no such disadvantage of using the anti-depressant during pregnancy but you need to make sure that you consult your doctor about using anti-depressants while you are pregnant. Some studies on the anti-depressants shows some risk of certain birth defects while other researchers have found no issue with these medicines.

**Anti-seizure Drugs:** Anti-seizure drugs have mild or no effect on pregnant women and newborns. But it is advised that you consult your doctor before you stop using this medicine. The seizures might be bad for the child than the drugs itself.

**High blood pressure medicine:** Some blood pressure medications are considered harmful during pregnancy and may cause issues for the infants. You need to make sure that you consult your doctor before using any blood pressure medicine.

**Blood Thinners:** Women who have issues related to blood clots and or have artificial heart valves are prescribed blood thinners. A blood thinner named Coumadin can cause issues for the fetus, and may also cause miscarriage so you need to make sure that you switch to other blood thinners when you are planning to conceive. Consult your medical practitioner for more information regarding blood thinners.

**Vitamin A:** Too much Vitamin A in the bloodstream of a pregnant woman can cause miscarriage and other complications when you are pregnant. You need to make sure that you eliminate the food items that contain Vitamin A from your diet when you are planning to use Vitamin A tablets.

**Birth Control Tablets:** There have been many reported cases of women who have become pregnant while they were using birth control pills. They either missed their dosage or were taking just a couple of tablets in the month. Birth control pills do not have any ill effect on child's birth.

**Using Nutritional Supplements**

Many women who love to use herbal medicine to treat their common ailments. Many herbal extracts or natural supplements are safe to use when you are pregnant, but you need to know that these supplements are not regulated by medical boards and may have some side effects. There have been fewer studies on the benefits of these herbal medications. These herbal medications are also known to interact with other medicines, so you should take caution when using this medicine. Herbal medications may cause miscarriage or uterine contractions and should be avoided when you are pregnant. Some herbal medications that are safe to use during pregnancy are blue cohosh, juniper berry, mistletoe, and goldenseal.

**Understanding The Need For Vaccination And Immunity**

Immunity helps people to stay healthy and free of infections. People are immune to diseases because of these two reasons. They received a shot that causes the body to develop antibodies. People also become immune to a disease because they have that disease before and their bodies have developed the antibodies to fight the infection.

The doctor will ask whether you have received the shot of rubella. They can take your blood sample and check whether you are immune to the rubella virus or not. If you are not immune to the rubella virus, they will recommend that you take a rubella shot at least three months before you are pregnant. No problems have been reported in babies whose mothers got pregnant before the three months are over. Most vaccinations are safe to use while pregnant.

Many people are immune to different infections such as poliomyelitis, mumps, and measles; your practitioner will not check for the immunity against these infections. These ailments are not considered harmful for the newborn and does have not adverse effect on the growth of the baby. Chickenpox has a small risk and the baby can get this infection from the mother. If you have never had chickenpox, you should tell this to the medical officer before you conceive.

Additionally, there has been a risk of the HIV infection, and you need to have an HIV test before planning to get pregnant. If you have been tested HIV positive, you need to take some medications during the pregnancy to ensure that the baby does not get the HIV . HPV virus has been known to affect the genitals of the females and cause issues such as cervical cancer and genital warts. A new vaccination has been introduced that can control human papillomavirus. You should ask your doctor about the virus and take a shot 30 days before you plan on pregnant.

**Stop Using Birth Control Methods**

If you are confused about how soon you can get pregnant after quitting the birth control, then the answer is simple. The time of conceiving after quitting birth control depends on the method you are using. Condoms and spermicides work for as long as you use them. Other hormone-based systems such as ortho-Evra take sufficient time to stop working in the system once you use them. It can take some months for the normal ovulatory system to restore.

There are no definite rules on when you should try to conceive after you have stopped using the birth control methods. You can start right away after you have stopped using the birth control methods. You need to understand that you have not resumed the monthly ovulation cycle and may face difficulty when you are trying to conceive. When you conceive before your ovulation cycles restarts, it will be difficult to know your exact due date. Start having sex when you are planning to conceive, and even if you don't get pregnant right away, you will at least have a good time.

**When To Worry About Infertility**

Subfertility or infertility is a problem that has been seen in many couples these days. People wait for a long time to become parents, and this has caused many healthy males and females to become infertile. One out of ten couples face many problems in becoming parents, and this ratio turns to one out of five in couples who are older than 35 years old. Age is never a problem when it comes to fertility. Many women in their 50s become mothers. It is very rare to see women of over 50 years old, becoming spontaneous mothers. When you have been trying to get pregnant for more than six months or a year and have been unsuccessful, then it is time that you should seek the help of a doctor.

Some women have experienced miscarriages and their partner may have low sperm count, these things can cause issues when you are trying to conceive. You should not get worried about any of these problems as reproductive systems become mature every year and you have more chances to become pregnant. Couples should seek fertility medications such as sperm injections and Vitro fertilization methods to have a baby.

## Timing Is Everything In Reproduction

We assume that everybody reading this book already knows about the process of reproduction. What people are most confused about is the way to make the process more effective and productive.

In this section, you will know the easiest way to get pregnant without any hassle. For this, you need to make sure that you understand the process of ovulation. Ovulation is the process in which the egg is released from the ovary, and this process is conducted every one cycle.

When the egg leaves the ovary, it spends more than two days sliding down in the fallopian tube and it reaches the womb. The egg fertilization will occur when the sperm will reach the egg in the first 24 hours from when it is released from the ovary.

Your job is to ensure that the egg meets the sperm ideally within 24 hours.

According to studies, the best time to have sex is approximately 12 hours before the egg is released from the ovaries. The sperms have a lifespan of about 24 to 48 hours and in rare cases, the sperm can fertilize eggs as much as after seven days. It should be noted that you will not get pregnant on your first try and you need to make sure that you repeat the sexual intercourse to increase the chance of your conceiving. There is an approx. Twenty-five percent chance to get pregnant every month. More than half of the couples who try to conceive gets possible result in the first four months. The success rate is increased to 93 percent in two years span. If you have been trying to get pregnant for more than a year and not getting adequate results, then you should get a fertility evaluation.

**Locating Ovulation**

Are you confused about when the ovulation happens? The phenomenon of ovulation happens rarely 14 days before you get your period. The usual menstrual cycle lasts for 28 days and the ovulation period will start after 14 days of your last period. If you have a menstrual cycle of 32 days, the ovulation period will come after 18 days of your previous period. If you are planning to conceive, you need to have sex more often during this time. This is to ensure that the sperm is in the right position. It is best to start having intercourse five days before the ovulation time and continue it for two to three days afterward. Now you will be wondering how many times you will have to have sex to get pregnant. Having sex once in two days is preferable. You need to know that many people believed that having sex daily can cause the sperm count to drop but this is an unfair assessment. The sperm count of men will drop after daily sex if they have less sperm count to start with.

**Checking the Body temperature**

Checking the body temperature at different times can help you to pinpoint the ovulation process. Checking your basal body temperature will surely help you to get pregnant easily. When you measure the body temperature, make sure that you check your temperature orally right after you wake up. It should be noted that the body temperature needs to be checked before you have something to eat or drink. The body temperature is at the lowest at the ovulation process. After the release of the LH hormone, your body temperature will be more than the baseline and will stay increased till you reach your period. It is best to buy the specialized basal body thermometers as they are easier to read and have larger grading as well.

The increase in the basal body temperature only indicates that the ovulation process has been completed in the body and it does not predict when you will ovulate. This will give you a rough idea about the ovulation cycle and you can be ready to have intercourse in the next ovulation cycle. These signals are sometimes hard to read but women can follow these patterns to ensure that they get pregnant easily. Remember that basal body temperature thermometers are not a hundred percent accurate and you should consult your doctor when you are planning to conceive.

**Make use of the ovulation predictor kit**

You can also use the ovulation predictor kit to monitor the LH surge. The ovulation predictor kit is used to predict the time of ovulation as opposed to the basal body temperature which tells you about the increase in the temperature when the ovulation has happened. The positive test on the ovulation kit will show that you are ready for ovulation and will also inform you about the mating cycles. One of the main issues with these kits is that they are fairly expensive. You will have to spend 20$ to 40$ per kit. You will have to spend a lot of money if you are planning to check for several cycles.

One other way to find out about the ovulation process is by testing the saliva. Due to the increased level of estrogen during the ovulation period, the saliva will show a crystalized pattern under a microscope. Both the saliva and urine tests are almost 98 percent accurate. The saliva testing kit will cost around 40$ and can be reused. Evaluating the cervical mucus is another way to check if you are ovulating. Your cervical mucus will turn to egg-white color when you are about the ovulate. This is a free method to Check Whether You Are Ovulating or Not.

## Always Use an Effective Approach

It is always recommended that the couples who are planning to conceive should stay relaxed and enjoy the process. You should not get anxious about the whole process, as this process won't happen in a heartbeat. You should stop using the birth control pills some months before you planning to get pregnant. In this way, you will be carefree when you are trying to conceive and you can enjoy the process without any worry whether you are pregnant or not. Having carefree sex will also calm your mind and you will not have any hurdle or tension in your mind. By this method, you will surely conceive way ahead of the time which will be a nice surprise for you. Here are some tips for enjoying the sex and conceiving easily. You need to quit smoking and marijuana and stay away from any illegal substance

- Make sure that you and your partner do not use any kind of commercial lubricants during sex. The K-Y jelly is known to contain the spermicides which may cause hurdles when you

are trying to conceive. You can use vegetable oil or olive oil for lubrication.
- If you drink more than three cups of coffee each day, this will decrease your chances of conceding.  Limiting your caffeine intake can help you to get pregnant easily.
- Women who are overweight need to stick to low-fat diet and work on a weight loss plan. If you are confused about how much weight you need to lose, take help from the dietician or a personal trainer.

# Chapter 2:

# Hurray! You Think You Are Pregnant

*You will learn*

---

*The Pregnancy Symptoms to Look Out For*

*Getting to Know If You Are Really Pregnant or Not*

*Finding the Right Doctor for Your Needs*

*Finding Your Due Date*

---

Congratulations, if you think that you are pregnant and you want to know about the changes that you will feel in the first few weeks. In this chapter, we will guide you regarding a few body signals that you feel in the first weeks of pregnancy. We will also provide advice to first-time moms to make sure that they are not spooked by this process and get a good start.

## The Right Signs of Pregnancy

Let's assume that you are pregnant and sperm has nestled in your womb's soft lining. So, how and when will you find out that you are expecting? The first sign that is observed by women is the "missed period". Your body will send you some signals – some even before your first missed period. You need to Pay attention to everybody changes.

**Baby, I am late!** You will know that you are pregnant when you didn't see your monthly flow. When you have missed the period, pregnancy test will definitely confirm that you are pregnant. Even when you are pregnant, you may feel some light bleeding which is due to the embryo attachment to the uterus.

**Your breast becomes bigger and softer!** You will probably notice that your breasts have become bigger at the early stages of your pregnancy and you should not be alarmed if this happens. This is one of the first signs that you will notice when you are pregnant. Women's estrogen levels rise when they are pregnant which causes an increase in the size of breasts.

**You will get food cravings!** Whatever you have heard about the increased appetite of pregnant women is true. You will crave pickles and pasta and will probably crave food items that are not your favorite. There is no explanation of why you feel the increased appetite and craving for these food items. As the studies show, this is nature's way to ensure that your body has the vital vitamins that are required during pregnancy. You will also crave starchy items such as potatoes and eating these foods will help you to store energy. This stored energy will help you in the later stages of pregnancy. You will need a lot of energy when the baby starts growing. Keeping all these things mind, you need to increase your food intake but make sure that you do not overeat. You will also feel thirsty most of the time when you are pregnant and drinking extra water will help your body fluids to be at the normal levels.

## Determining If You Are Pregnant

When a woman is trying to conceive, there is a constant battle in the mind of whether you are pregnant or not. You do not have to go to the doctor to find out that you are pregnant, there are many self-tests that you can do at home which will tell you exactly if you are pregnant or not. The generic home urine test can help you to know if you are pregnant or not. These tests are almost accurate for most people. The doctor will either test your blood or urine to know if you are pregnant or not. The test conducted by the doctors is more authentic than the home urine tests.

**Do-it-yourself Test for Answers**

Women usually conduct home tests when they have missed their period or when they have food cravings. Most women try to find the answer to their pregnancy at home because they do not want to visit the doctor just yet. You can visit the nearest drug store and buy a pregnancy test kit to know whether you are pregnant or not. These tests will check the human chorionic gonadotropin in your urine and will let you know if you are pregnant or not. You need to know that these tests are not accurate and can show a positive result when you have missed your period by a day. The best time to use these home tests is about 2 weeks after conception. These tests will not always show the right result. If you see the negative result but feel that you are pregnant, you should retake the test in a week or visit your doctor.

**Visiting the Doctor for Answers**

When you visit the doctor and tell them about the positive result in the home pregnancy kit, they will surely conduct another test at their hospital to ensure if you are really pregnant. It is up to the doctor to choose either the blood or urine test to test for pregnancy.

In a blood pregnancy test, the doctor will check the human chorionic gonadotropin in the blood. There are two ways to conduct this test – the doctor can either do a qualitative test which will show the positive or negative result or the doctor can choose to find the actual measurement of the chg. in the blood with the help of a quantitative test. The selection of the test will generally depend on the symptoms you are having. The doctor will also analyze your medical history before choosing a test type. The blood pregnancy test can come positive even if you are seeing negative results in the urine test.

## Finding the Right Doctor

Finding the right doctor when you are pregnant is very important and this is a decision that you do not want to take lightly. Both parents should be part of this decision. You might be comfortable with your old doctor till now but with your new and complicated situation, you need to make sure that you find the practitioner that is sync with your condition. Pregnancy doctor is someone that you feel safe with. Do not be confused about the selection of the new healthcare practitioner as this section will address all your concerns and provide important information about the selection process.

### Understand Different Options

There are different kinds of professionals that can help you get through this phase. You need to make sure that you choose the healthcare provider which you feel comfortable with. These are the four main types of healthcare providers that you will come across:

**Midwife-Nurse:** This is a certified medical officer who is allowed to stay with the pregnant women and can also perform deliveries. They possess a full license and these nurses will communicate with different doctors and experts to ensure no complications occur. A specialist is always on-call if any complication arises.

**Family Practice Physician:** This is the medical professional that provides basic health care for women, men, and children. This type of medical professional is certified in family medicine. This doctor will help you in the first few months of your pregnancy and will recommend you to a gynecologist at the time of delivery.

**Maternal-fetal medicine doctor:** This medical professional has completed two to three years of high-risk pregnancy cases and can advise you regarding all the aspects of the pregnancy. Most of the maternal-fetal medicine specialists work as medical specialists and some also offer their services in high-risk delivery cases.

**Gynecologist:** This is the type of doctor who has a four-year specialization in the field of pregnancy. They are well-versed in all the medicines and latest medical practices of women's health. A gynecologist is certified with the American Board of Obstetrics and Gynecology.

Many people believe that pregnancy lasts for nine months but a healthy baby is delivered in over 40 weeks. They make more than nine months so the doctor will probably discuss all the medicine and timeline in terms of weeks. This count will generally start at least two weeks before you conceive. When the doctor says that you are fifteen weeks pregnant, this states that your fetus is only thirteen weeks old.

A woman will not know whether her pregnancy is at high risk right at the start. There is no clear answer to the high-risk pregnancy and no specific way to determine the outcome of the delivery in the state. There are some situations that can increase the risk at the time of delivery. Some conditions that you should be aware of are blood disorders, multiple fetuses, history of miscarriage, bleeding, infections and high blood pressure. You need to remember that the nurse-midwife is not equipped for dealing with these complications and you should see a gynecologist if you are faced with these above-mentioned conditions.

## Right Questions to Ask Before You Make A Decision

You need to make sure that you do a thorough background check and ask the right questions before you make a final decision regarding the medical professional. You need to hire a person who has relevant experience in the field. Asking these simple questions will help you gauge the knowledge of the medical professional.

Should I be confident that I have made the right choice? It is not only the doctor that you need to vet when you are choosing the healthcare professional. The establishment and the people who work with the doctor also plays a vital role in the pregnancy. Being pregnant is an important milestone in your life and you will need to work with the people who you feel comfortable with. While some women choose to have a detailed test in all the phases, there are some women who like to keep this process in a low-key. Your mental approach regarding your general health will play an important role in the selection of the doctor.

How many medical professionals will you have to deal with in this process? There are many medical officers who like to work alone with the patients and there are some who like to work with other professionals in the same case. In this way, they can rotate shifts and work with others to achieve success. When you are making the selection of the medical professional, ask them whether they will handle your case on their own or will take help from other doctors. Generally, a woman needs to have different medical professionals while they are pregnant. You should also inquire about the emergencies on holidays and after-hours.

Does this practitioner have links with other doctors in this field? You need to be sure that the medical professional can refer you to other doctors if something comes up. If you ever need help with the care of the infant, will the doctor be able to refer you to the physician who specializes in child care?

Is insurance enough to cover my medical bills? Managed care is an important part of many citizens and you need to inquire if your medical insurance will cover the bills of the physician you have selected. There are some hospitals that will also allow you to use the out-of-network physicians and you can pay their bills separately.

What hospital is the doctor working with? If you do not have any complications with your pregnancy, any medical office or hospital will be fine. If there are chances of complications, you need to make sure that you choose the medical professional who works with a hospital that has nursing stations and other facilities. If the child is born before the due date, the hospital should be able to cater for the needs of the infant.

**Finding Your Due Date**

There are only 1 in 20 women who give delivery on their due date – the other women deliver two to three weeks before the due date and some even deliver after the due date. Pinpointing the due date will help you to complete the tests during pregnancy and make sure that all the procedures are completed in due time. When the due date is calculated, the doctors will also feel safe measuring the growth of the baby.

From the first day of the last menstrual period – the pregnancy will last anywhere between 38 to 40 weeks. The due date is known as the estimated date of confinement and this is the date when the hospital prepares for your delivery. You can use professional help to make sure that you find the exact due date. You can also use these simple tips to find your due date. If your menstrual cycle lasts for 28 days, you can subtract three months and add seven days to find out your due date. If you have your last period in July, your due date will be somewhere in April. If your menstrual period is more than 28 days, do not worry you can easily find out your due date.

If you do not remember the date of your last menstrual cycle, a simple ultrasound in the first few weeks of pregnancy will help you know the due date. Ultrasound which is conducted in the first trimester will provide a good idea of the due date than the second and third trimester one.

## Some Old Pregnancy Myths That You Need to Know

Pregnancy has a specific persona. A large number of ladies have experienced it, yet foreseeing in detail what any one's experience will resemble is troublesome. Maybe that is the reason such a significant number of legends have shaped throughout the hundreds of years, the vast majority of which is intended to predict the mysterious future. Here are twelve stories that are actually only nonsense:

The Mysterious Umbilical Cord Movement Myth: If a pregnant lady lifts her hands over her head, she will stifle the child. Individuals used to think (and, oh dear, some still accept) that the mother's development could make the child become tangled in the umbilical rope; however, that is simply false.

The Old Heartburn Myth: If a pregnant lady encounters indigestion, her child will have a full head of hair. Essentially false, few babies have hair; some don't. Most lose everything inside half a month, at any rate.

The Curse Myth: Anyone who denies a pregnant lady the nourishment that she hungers for will get a pen in his eye. This fantasy doesn't imply that somebody who remains between a pregnant lady and her craving is getting into trouble. This is a myth that is completely false.

The Heart Rate Myth: If the fetal pulse is quick, the infant is a young lady, and if the pulse is moderate, the infant is a kid. Restorative inquiries about really investigated this fantasy. They found a slight contrast between the normal pulse of young men and that of young ladies, however, it wasn't huge enough to make pulse an exact indicator of sex.

The Ugly Stick Myth: If a pregnant lady sees something appalling or awful, she will have a terrible child. How could this be valid? There's nothing of the sort as an appalling child!

The Java Myth: If an infant is brought into the world with bistro au lait spots (light-darker skin pigmentations), the mother drank an excess of espresso or had unfulfilled yearnings during her pregnancy. Not a chance.

The Ultrasound Tells All Myth: Ultrasound can generally tell the infant's sex. No, not generally. Frequently, by around 18 to 20 weeks of incubation, seeing an embryo's genitalia on ultrasound is conceivable. Be that as it may, having the option to decide the child's sex relies upon whether the infant is in the position to give you a decent view. Once in a while the sonographer can't see between the uncooperative child's legs and in this manner can't decide the sex. Once in a while, as well, the sonographer might not be right, particularly if the ultrasound is done from the get-go in the pregnancy. So even though you can discover the child's sex through ultrasound much of the time, it's not 100 percent ensured.

The Round Face Myth: If a pregnant lady puts on weight in her face, the infant is a young lady. What's more, the end product fantasy says that if a lady puts on weight in her butt, the infant is a kid. Neither one of the statements is valid, clearly enough. The child's sex has no impact whatsoever in transit the mother stores fat. Another apparently related legend is that if the mother's nose starts to develop and extend, the infant is a young lady. The supposed thinking here is that a little girl consistently takes her mom's magnificence. Peculiar idea — and very false.

The Belly Shape Myth: If a pregnant woman's stomach is round, the infant is a young lady, and if the lady's midsection is more projectile like, it's a kid. Don't worry about it. Midsection shape varies from lady to lady, yet the kid's sex has nothing to do with it.

The Moon Maid Myth: This one holds that more ladies start giving birth during a full moon. Albeit many work and conveyance staff demand that the work floor is busier during a full moon (police say their area houses are livelier at that point, as well), the logical information simply doesn't bolster the thought.

The Great Sex Myth: Having enthusiastic sex expedites work. What got you into this chaos will likewise get you out? That is simply unrealistic reasoning, however, feel free to attempt it (on the off chance that you feel like it when you're nine months pregnant). It's probably going to merit the exertion.

# Chapter 3:
# Prepare Yourself for Pregnancy

*You will learn*

---

*What is a parental visit?*

*Coping with the body and mind changes*

*Changing the lifestyle for a healthy pregnancy*

---

When you are pregnant, you will see a lot of changes in your body and some will even affect your day-to-day life but you will need to complete all the daily chores as life won't stop. What are some of the changes that you will feel when you are pregnant? What lifestyle changes do you need to make when you are pregnant? There are many things that you need to understand and learn and, in this chapter, we will try to cover all these topics and make you prepare you for the pregnancy journey. You will be confused about whether you should drink or smoke, how often do you need to visit the doctor. Do not worry as all these topics will be discussed here in detail.

All the issues highlighted in this book are for information purposes. You need to trust the judgment of the doctor and make sure that you discuss all these issues with your doctor and follow these instructions to ensure safe delivery. You need to understand that your daily life will be changed and the sooner you adjust to your new diet, and overall health problem, the better it will be.

## Plan Parental Visit

When you have a positive pregnancy test, your new life will begin. This is the time when you think about the challenges that lie ahead and how you can manage your overall life and pregnancy. With the help of the tips that you have read in chapter 2, you will be able to find the right medical officer for you. You can either visit the family doctor for the blood or urine test to confirm the news or you can visit the gynecologist for the advice and the first parental visit. The decision boils down to your medical history and your approach to the pregnancy. When you have not had a preconception visit then you need to tell the doctor about the medications that you are using. You need to make sure that you take the right amount of vitamin dose when you are pregnant and for this, you can also ask for help from the pharmacist. Many things will remain common during the pregnancy such as checking the baby's heartbeat, the urine test and checking the blood pressure of the mother and more information will be provided by the healthcare professional during the first parental visit.

The parental visits are not fixed for every patient. When you have a complicated pregnancy, your doctor will ask you to come more frequently for checkups and other tests. There is no restriction on parental visits. If you are planning a vacation or need to make a trip, you need to tell your doctor about it and they will adjust the parental visit. When you have a normal pregnancy, rescheduling the parental visit is not a problem. You need to know that there are some tests that are mandatory and you cannot skip them. Make sure the missed appointments do not affect the test schedule.

The parental visit will differ for each woman and they also depend on the doctor's working style and ethics. There are some laboratory tests and pregnancy examinations that are vital during pregnancy. Some tests that you can expect during the parental visits are:

**The body weight and blood pressure:** The nurse will check your blood pressure and body weight on each parental visit. This will help the doctor to analyze your pregnancy and the growth of the baby.

**Urine Sample:** The doctor will check the glucose level and protein in the urine so that they can analyze your health. This will also let them know about problems such as diabetes and preeclampsia. The urine sample will also let the doctor know about any urinary tract infection that you might have.

**Measuring the fundal height:** When you are 14 to 16 weeks pregnant, the doctor will test your fundal height as well. The doctor will use the measuring tape to measure the size of your uterus. This will let them know about the growth of the baby and whether your body is responding correctly to the baby's growth. The fundal height is the measurement from the top of the pubic bone to the top of the uterus.

**The doctor will listen to the baby's heartbeat:** The average heartbeat of a baby is 120 to 160 bpm. The doctors will use a Doppler machine to hear and count the heartbeats of the baby. The heartbeat of the baby can be felt after 8 to 9 weeks with this method and in some rare cases, the heartbeat is not clearly heard until 12 weeks of pregnancy.

## Prepare Yourself for Emotional Changes

While being pregnant, you will see many emotional and physical changes in yourself. Some common changes that you will feel are muscle cramps, mood swings, and elevated stress. You may have felt these changes in the past but when you are pregnant, you will fell these changes in high intensity. In this section, you will understand how these changes will prevail with your lifestyle and how you can manage them during pregnancy. It is important that you let your partner, and your family read this section so that they can understand what your body and mind are going through.

**Increased Mood Swings**

Stress is the first thing that you are going to notice when you are pregnant. The women who suffer from premenstrual syndrome understand how stress affects their mind when their body is going through different changes. The hormone shifts that happen during pregnancy are the most severe that a woman has to face in their entire life. It is common to see pregnant women snap at the smallest of things and lose their temper. Women feel more fatigue during the pregnancy and this fatigue can increase the stress that they face. The women also face the tension of whether their baby will be healthy or not and this stress also affects their body and increase the mood swings.

You need to understand that mood swings are common when you are pregnant and you should try to stay as relaxed as possible. You are not the only woman that is suffering from mood swings and you should make your friends and family understand this fact.

The mood swings will be severe in the first 12 weeks as the body will be coping with the new changes. You should not get rattled when you lose anything or missed an appointment. Elevated stress and mood swings are common so be prepared for it. You simply need to close your eyes when you have a tantrum of mood swings and let the feeling pass.

**Prepare for Leg Cramps**

Your body will take time to adjust with the additional weight and you will feel frequent leg cramps during your pregnancy. The leg cramps will worsen as the months' pass. The sudden tightening of the muscles also increases these leg cramps. The lack of fluids in the body and decreased movement are the main reasons behind these leg cramps. In older times, the doctor thought the deficiency of calcium and potassium in the body was the main cause of the leg cramps but after thorough research in this department, it was found out that this is not the case with many women. However, taking oral vitamins may decrease the effects of leg cramps.

If you are worried about the leg cramps, use these simple tips to decrease their pain. You can apply heat to the calves and increase your water intake to take care of the cramps. You also need to move the legs in order to keep the blood flowing and this will reduce the leg cramps. Stretching your legs and toes can also help you to reduce muscle cramps. You can ask your partner for a leg massage and also take a short walk to decrease the cramps.

**Vaginal discharge**

When you are pregnant, the vaginal discharge will increase substantially. The vaginal discharge during the pregnancy will be of white color and will be odorless. Due to the additional discharge, many women need to wear thin panty liners. If the discharge is of yellow or green color, you need to make sure that you let the doctor know. Apart from this, you also need to tell the doctor if you are getting rashes near the vagina. This is not an emergency but the doctor needs to know this so that they can plan their next step. A woman can get a vaginal infection during pregnancy and with the elevated levels of estrogen in the body, you may get yeast infection as well. You may need to use the over-the-counter medication to counter the infections.

**Increased Backaches**

Backaches are very common during pregnancy and they mostly happen in the latter part of the pregnancy. When you are pregnant, there is a shift in your center of gravity and this causes back pain. When the baby grows, there is a change in the curvature of the body and the spine and this can also lead to backaches. You can tackle this back pain by increasing your movement and also increasing the water intake. Apart from this, there is a pregnancy girdle that you can use to decrease the back pain.

Women experience different types of backaches. Some women will feel pain in the upper part of the back and others will experience pain in the lower back which extends to the legs. You may also feel some numbness in the body which is due to the increased stress on the sciatic nerve. You can relieve your body from numbness by bed rest and special exercises.

**Coping with Stress**

Many women think that stress affects the pregnancy but there are no reports where stress has tweaked the growth of the baby. Stress is a very complicated concept and every person has their way of dealing with stress. No one can accurately measure the effect of stress and how the increases stress levels change the hormones in the body. Doctors suggest that you need to learn to control the stress when you are pregnant as chronic stress can lead to increased blood pressure and preterm labor issues in women who are pregnant.

# How Medications, Drugs, And Alcohol Affect Your Body

Alcohol and recreational drugs are dangerous for the baby. They can enter the placenta and harm the baby's growth. Apart from these, you also need to know that many medicines can pass through the placenta. While some are harmless, there are some medications that you should avoid when you are pregnant. It is important that you do not use any medication without prior consultation with your doctor.

**Medications:**

When you are pregnant, you will face issues such as headache and heartburn and you will feel the unwillingness to take medications. The main question that you need to address is whether these medications will have any side effects and how you will be able to cater to the increased need of your body. There are many women who are afraid to take the medication as they fear for the safety of their babies. You need to understand that most medications are harmless when you are pregnant. When you visit the doctor for the first parental visit, make sure that you discuss all medications you have been taking with your doctor. If you are getting treated for a disease, tell your doctor that you are pregnant so that the medication can be adjusted according to your needs.

It is advised that you should not stop taking medications without consulting your doctor. You also nccd to discuss if you are planning to change the dosage. There are some medications that are labeled "not safe for women in pregnancy". There are fewer studies of pregnant women and whenever you are confused about any medication, take advice from a qualified medical officer. Different medical officers might have different opinions regarding medicine. Do not get surprised after listening to the different opinions of the doctors. We have discussed the medications that might have an adverse effect on the child's growth in the previous chapters so take extra care when it comes to medication.

**Smoking**

Everyone knows that smoking is hazardous to the health. At the point when you smoke, you risk creating lung malignant growth, emphysema, and coronary illness, among different sicknesses. During pregnancy, be that as it may, smoking postures dangers to your infant too.

The carbon monoxide in tobacco smoke diminishes the measure of oxygen that your developing infant gets, and nicotine reduces bloodstream to the baby. Thus, ladies who smoke stand an expanded possibility of conveying babies with low birth weight, which may mean progressively medicinal issues for the infant. Truth be told, babies destined to smokers are required to gauge a half-pound less, by and large, than those destined to nonsmokers. The careful distinction in birth weight relies on how much the mother smokes. Used smoke is additionally a hazard.

Notwithstanding low birth weight, smoking during pregnancy is related to a more serious danger of preterm conveyance, unsuccessful labor, placenta previa, placental suddenness), preterm crack of the amniotic films and even unexpected newborn child demise disorder (SIDS) after the infant is conceived.

Stopping smoking can be very troublesome. In any case, remember that even cutting back on the number of cigarettes you smoke is valuable to your infant (and yourself).

On the off chance that you quit smoking during the initial three months you're pregnant, give your-self a congratulatory gesture and be consoled that your infant is probably going to be conceived at an ordinary weight and have fewer medical problems.

A few ladies use nicotine patches, gum, capsules, or inhalers to assist them with kicking the addiction. The nicotine from these items can pass in the bloodstream and can affect the growth of the unborn child. When you use these patches, the carbon monoxide and different poisons in tobacco smoke are wiped out. The American College of Obstetrics and Gynecology prescribes that nicotine substitutions, for example, these might be utilized when nonpharmacologic medicines have fizzled. The aggregate sum of nicotine consumed from the irregular utilization of the gum or inhalers might not be exactly the sum from the fix, which is utilized constantly.

The consequences for fetal advancement with the utilization of bupropion (Zyban or Wellbutrin) haven't been widely examined, yet one well-planned examination demonstrated that pregnant smokers getting bupropion were substantially more liable to stop than those not taking the drug.

**Drinking liquor**

Obviously, pregnant ladies who use liquor put their infants in danger of fetal liquor disorder, which envelops a wide assortment of birth absconds (counting development issues, heart deserts, mental hindrance, or variations from the norm of the face or appendages). The debate emerges because therapeutic science hasn't characterized a flat out the safe degree of liquor consumption during pregnancy. Logical information shows that day by day drinking and substantial hard-core boozing can prompt genuine inconveniences, albeit little data is accessible about periodic drinking. The American College of Obstetricians and Gynecologists and the Food and Drug Administration prescribe maintaining a strategic distance from any measure of liquor.

If you figure you may have a drinking issue, don't feel awkward conversing with your specialist about it. Exceptional polls are accessible to enable your primary care physician to distinguish whether your drinking is unreasonable enough to represent a hazard to you and the baby. On the off chance that you figure you may have an issue, examining this survey with your professional is pivotal to your child's wellbeing — and yours.

**Utilizing recreational/unlawful medications**

Numerous studies have assessed the impacts of medication use during pregnancy. However, the investigations can be confounding because they will in general protuberance a wide range of medication clients together, paying little respect to which drugs they use and the amount they use. The mother's way of life likewise impacts the level of hazard to the child, which confounds the data significantly more. For instance, ladies who misuse drugs are bound to be malnourished than other ladies, they are common of lower financial status, and they endure a higher frequency of explicitly transmitted ailments. Every one of these elements, autonomous of and added to sedate use, can mess up your pregnancy and for your infant.

## Making Lifestyle Changes

Your way of life unavoidably changes during your pregnancy. You may ponder whether it's still alright to accomplish a portion of the things you may have indulged in before you were pregnant. This area gives data on exercises, for example, regardless of whether you can go into saunas and hot tubs, whether you can travel, and whether you can keep working.

### Spoiling yourself with excellence medicines

At the point when your companions and family members hear that you're pregnant, they'll most likely disclose to you how excellent you look or what a dazzling maternal sparkle you have. Also, you may feel progressively wonderful, as well, a few ladies feel the accurate inverse. You may find that you're not content with the physical changes that are going on to your body. In any case, you're similar to the vast majority of our patients, and you may wonder how these changes will affect life after pregnancy. In this segment, we go over them individually and let you think about any potential dangers:

Botox: The wellbeing of Botox treatment during pregnancy and breastfeeding is obscure. Our recommendation? Appreciate the excellence from your pregnancy gleam while you're pregnant, and hang tight for the Botox.

Chemical strips: Alpha-hydroxy acids are the fundamental fixings in substance strips. The synthetic compounds work topically, however modest quantities are retained into your framework. We haven't found any information on whether synthetic strips are protected during pregnancy. They're most likely alright, yet first talk about it with your expert.

Facials: You may see that your composition has changed in the course of recent months. Some of the time pregnancy hormones can unleash destruction on your skin. Facials could possibly help. Be that as it may, feel free to have one at any rate, on the off chance that just to appreciate an opportunity to take a load off! (See the former remarks about synthetic strips.)

Injectable fillers: Injectable skin fillers are utilized to smooth wrinkles and make lips fuller. Frequently they're made with collagen or hyaluronic acid. Nothing more than bad memory information right now exists reporting the wellbeing of fillers during pregnancy. Fortunately, the liquid maintenance of pregnancy may reduce the wrinkles in any case!

Hair colors: Using hair colors during pregnancy is likely fine. No proof recommends that hair colors cause birth imperfections or premature delivery. Quite a while back, some of them contained formaldehyde and other conceivably perilous synthetic substances that could hurt a child. Yet, the more current colors don't contain these synthetic substances. Specialists will, in general, differ on this issue. Your professional may instruct you to adhere to vegetable hair colors during pregnancy, while your companion's specialist may disclose to her that coloring her hair is fine.

Manicures and pedicures: Another as often as possible posed inquiry is: "Would I be able to have a nail treatment/pedicure or have nail tips or acrylic nails set while I'm pregnant?" Again, the appropriate response is yes. Sound judgment proposes that you go to a legitimate salon where the hardware is appropriately cleaned and the zone is all around ventilated.

Hair waxing: Waxing legs or the two-piece line includes applying a warmed wax arrangement topically and afterward evacuating it alongside the hair. Nothing in the wax arrangements can prompt issues for the child. Ward off waxing while you're pregnant to assist you with staying lighthearted and without hair.

Massages: Massages are fine, and you'll see that many back-rub advisors offer extraordinary pregnancy kneads planned for pleasing your pregnant tummy. Some utilization unique tables with the inside cut out so you can easily lie face down, particularly in the last some portion of the pregnancy.

Permanents: No logical proof proposes that the synthetic concoctions in hair permanents are destructive to the creating child. These arrangements generally contain huge measures of smelling salts, be that as it may, so for your own wellbeing, use them in well-ventilated zones.

Laser hair evacuation: The laser utilized for hair expulsion works by transmit-ting warmth to the hair follicle and halting hair regrowth. Regularly soporific creams are applied to the skin first to diminish torment. In spite of the fact that we couldn't discover explicit information on laser hair evacuation during pregnancy, we are aware of no explanation that this treatment, which is applied locally, should make any issue the child.

Thermal reconditioning: Thermal reconditioning, otherwise called the Japanese fixing procedure, is a genuinely new strategy to fix hair forever. The procedure includes applying an assortment of synthetic compounds and conditioners to the hair, and afterward utilizing a level iron to for all time fix the hair. No logical research has examined this system in pregnancy. A portion of the synthetic compounds utilized is like those utilized for perming hair. The primary concern: Thermal reconditioning is likely alright during pregnancy, yet we are aware of no conclusive information.

**Using Steam Rooms, Saunas and Hot Tubs While Pregnant**

Utilizing hot tubs or steam rooms when you're pregnant can be dangerous as a result of the high temperatures included. In research facility creatures, presentation to elevated levels of warmth during pregnancy has been known to cause birth imperfections or premature delivery. Studies including people propose that pregnant ladies whose center internal heat levels rise essentially during long early stretches of pregnancy may stand an expanded danger of unnatural birth cycle or having babies with neural cylinder surrenders (spina bifida, for instance).

Nonetheless, issues ordinarily happen just if the mother's center temperature transcends 102 degrees Fahrenheit (or around 39 degrees Celsius) for over ten minutes during the initial seven weeks of her pregnancy. By and large, absorbing a warm, relieving shower is fine during pregnancy. Simply ensure that the water temperature isn't unreasonably high, for the reasons just referenced.

It is recommended that after the principal trimester, once in a while utilizing hot tubs, saunas, and steam spaces for under ten minutes is likely alright. Notwithstanding, make sure to drink a lot of liquids to maintain a strategic distance from lack of hydration.

**Voyaging**

The primary potential issue with going during pregnancy is that it puts separation among you and your pre-birth care supplier. In case you're near your due date or if your pregnancy is viewed as high-chance, you most likely shouldn't go a long way from home. Your choice to travel, however, relies upon what the hazard factors really are. If you have diabetes yet, it's all around controlled, going out traveling is most likely alright. Be that as it may, in case you're pregnant with triplets, venturing out to Timbuktu most likely is certifiably not a smart thought. On the off chance that your pregnancy is uncomplicated, travel during the principal, second, and early third trimesters are normally alright.

Going via vehicle represents no unique hazard, besides necessitating that you sit in one place for quite a while. On long outings, stop each couple of hours to get out and stroll around a piece. Wear your safety belt and shoulder tie; they guard you, and they won't hurt the child, regardless of whether you're in a mishap. The amniotic liquid encompassing the embryo fills in as a pad against any tightening from the lap belt. Not wearing restrictions unmistakably represents a more serious hazard; thinks about the show that the main source of fetal passing in car crashes is the demise of the mother. Wear your safety belt underneath your stomach area, not above it, and keep the shoulder lash in its typical position.

Most aircraft enable ladies to fly If they're under 36 weeks pregnant, however, you might need to convey a note from your expert demonstrating that she sees no therapeutic motivation behind why you shouldn't fly. Flying is impeccably sheltered, particularly on the off chance that you take two or three precautionary measures:

Get up from your seat at times during long flights and stroll around the plane. Drawn out times of sitting can make blood pool in your legs. Strolling around props your dissemination up.

Carry a water bottle with you and drink water often. Plane air is in every case exceptionally dry. (A pilot once revealed to us that the relative stickiness in planes is commonly lower than in the Sahara Desert. Planes can't convey enough water to keep the moistness up, because the additional water would include an excess of payload weight.) Because plane air is so dry, you can without much of a stretch become got dried out during long flights.

Drinking additional water likewise guarantees that you get up every now and again to go to the bathroom, which shields the blood from pooling in your legs.

You don't have to stress over air terminal metal identifiers — or some other metal indicators — because they don't utilize ionizing radiation. (The transport line that conveys your gear after you check it in uses ionizing radiation, notwithstanding, so we don't prescribe that you climb onto the counter and send yourself through that machine.)

In case you're inclined to queasiness and have discovered Dramamine supportive before, utilizing it in ordinary portions while you're pregnant is alright.

On the off chance that you intend to visit tropical nations, where a few infections are especially pervasive, you might need to be inoculated before you go. In any case, check with your PCP to see whether any immunizations you're thinking about are sheltered to have during pregnancy.

**Getting dental consideration**

A great many people see their dental specialist for routine cleanings each 6 to a year, which implies you'll likely need to visit your dental specialist in any event once during your pregnancy. Pregnancy itself shouldn't influence your dental wellbeing. You would prefer not to maintain a strategic distance from the dental specialist because dismissed depressions can get contaminated, which is even more motivation to see your dental specialist when you're pregnant. Some ongoing investigations have demonstrated that pregnant ladies who experience the ill effects of periodontal ailment, which is disease and irritation of the gums, are at a higher hazard for conveying little or untimely children. This finding is one more explanation behind making great oral cleanliness a need.

Pregnancy makes an expansion in the bloodstream the gums. Truth be told, about a portion of every single pregnant lady build up a condition called pregnancy gum disease, which is just blushing of the gums brought about by this expanded bloodstream. In this condition, gums tend to drain effectively, so attempt to be delicate when you brush and floss your teeth.

For those of you who need whiter and more splendid teeth, a lot of items are accessible, including brightening toothpaste and over-the-counter gels, strips, brightening frameworks, and plate. Albeit most are as often as possible utilized during pregnancy, no huge investigations archive the security of such medications.

Brightening toothpaste assists in evacuating the surfacing stains without any dye. There is no motivation to think they are an issue. Over-the-counter brightening strips, gels, and brightening frameworks are peroxide-based and haven't been explicitly contemplated in pregnancy. Be that as it may, the security of peroxide can be suggested from different examinations. In one such examination, pregnant rodents were sustained up to 10 percent hydrogen peroxide in their eating routine and no issues were distinguished in their posterity. Additionally, when tried as a segment in hair colors, peroxide wasn't found to cause birth absconds. With in-office dying, the professional applies the brightening item to the teeth, and utilizations heat as well as a laser to enliven the procedure. Numerous dental specialists don't play out these methods on pregnant ladies since they haven't been well-contemplated. On the brilliant side, seeing your dental specialist for cleaning advances great cleanliness, yet additionally evacuates surface stains and leaves you with a more brilliant grin.

On the off chance that you need routine dental work — pits filled, teeth pulled, crowns put — don't stress. Nearby anesthesia and most agony meds are sheltered. A few dental specialists additionally suggest anti-infection agents during dental systems. Most anti-infection agents that dental specialists prescribe are additionally protected during pregnancy; however, you should check with your pre-birth care supplier to ensure. Indeed, even dental X-beams represent no critical issue for the baby, up to a lead "cover" or shield is set over the midriff.

**Engaging in Sexual Relations**

For most couples, engaging in sexual relations during pregnancy is flawlessly sheltered. Indeed, a few couples find that sex during pregnancy is shockingly better than previously. Be that as it may, you may have a few issues to consider.

In the main portion of pregnancy, sex can typically proceed as before because your body hasn't changed that perceptibly. You may see that your bosoms are especially delicate to the touch, or considerably delicate. Afterward, as the uterus develops, some sexual positions become progressively troublesome. You and your partner may see that you have as somewhat inventive to make things work. On the off chance that you find that intercourse is excessively awkward, different types of sexual delight may work better for you and your partner.

Numerous ladies ask us in the case of having intercourse toward the finish of pregnancy is alright, regardless of whether the cervix is a smidgen expanded. Having intercourse at that point is consummately fine as long as your films haven't cracked (your water hasn't broken).

Stay away from intercourse in case you're at a high hazard for preterm work or If you have placenta previa.

Another significant perspective to consider is how every one of you feels mentally about engaging in sexual relations during pregnancy. Like a few ladies, you may find that your charisma or sex drive has expanded. Frequently, you may find that you have striking sexual dreams and that climax itself is elevated. Then again, you may find that your enthusiasm for sex is short of what it was before you got pregnant. You may feel less appealing on account of the physical changes that have occurred, which is impeccably typical. Your partner may likewise encounter changes in his craving for sex because of the energy and typical anxiety that accompanies being a dad and because of (unwarranted) feelings of trepidation that intercourse will hurt the infant or that the child will find some way or another realize what mother and father are doing.

## Working When You Are Pregnant

In the course of the last 50 years, the quantity of ladies who work outside the home has relentlessly expanded. Presently more than 75 percent of pregnant ladies' work during the third trimester, and the greater part works inside half a month of conveyance. Numerous ladies locate that working until the finish of pregnancy keeps them glad and involved and causes them not to concentrate on the distresses. Also, numerous ladies don't have a decision — they might be the principle to pay suppliers for their families and their vocations are a top need. Albeit more often than not working all through pregnancy doesn't cause any issues for the child, there can be a few special cases.

Worry in pregnancy, regardless of whether identified with work or to home circumstances, isn't well-examined. A few specialists accept that very elevated levels of pressure may expand the danger of creating preeclampsia or preterm work, albeit no investigation has affirmed this hazard. Surprising pressure may build your danger of post-birth anxiety. An excessive amount of pressure clearly isn't useful for anybody. Do whatever you can to diminish the worry in your life and chat with your expert If you find you're getting diligently blue or on edge.

**Thinking about work-related risks**

Possibly your activity requires insignificant standing or strolling, enables you to work standard hours, and never worries you. If that is the situation, and If you have no past therapeutic issues, you may similarly also skirt this segment (and let us recognize what your activity is!). In any case, in case you're similar to all of us, read on.

Occupations that are physically requesting can be hazardous. Most employments fall someplace in the middle of inactive and requesting, however, and still, at the end of the day, the measure of pressure fluctuates as per the person. If your pregnancy continues without complexities, you most likely can keep on stirring until conveyance. In any case, a few intricacies that may emerge during pregnancy may make diminishing your remaining burden or halting work by and large prudent.

For instance, on the off chance that you create preterm work, your specialist will undoubtedly encourage you to quit working. Different conditions that may warrant a decrease in the physical movement are hypertension or issues with the infant's development.

On the off chance that you work at a work station, you may ponder whether you're being presented to anything hurtful. In any case, you have no compelling reason to stress — no proof proposes that the electromagnetic fields that work stations emanate are an issue.

A few consider proposing that ladies who have occupations related to physically requesting obligations, for example, truly difficult work, physical work, or noteworthy physical effort, might be at a somewhat higher danger of preterm birth, hypertension, preeclampsia, or little for-gestational-age babies. Then again, long working hours weren't found to expand the odds for unexpected labor. Different think about have additionally demonstrated that occupations in which delayed standing is required (over eight hours every day) were related with a more noteworthy possibility for back and foot torment, circulatory issues, and a marginally expanded danger of preterm birth. The uplifting news: The utilization of help hose, even though not especially appealing, is useful in diminishing varicose veins.

Keep in mind that your wellbeing and the infant's wellbeing are the most elevated need. Try not to feel that you're a weakling since you need to take care of your pregnancy. A few ladies accept that If they whine about specific indications or invest significant energy from a bustling calendar to eat or go to the washroom, they will collect the dissatisfaction with their bosses at work. Try not to give yourself a chance to feel regretful about your exceptional needs during this time, and don't give workers a chance to make you disregard any abnormal indications. If you need a break to manage complexities, take it, and don't feel terrible about it. Individuals who have never been pregnant don't completely comprehend the physical strains you're managing.

**Getting pregnant and the law**

Set aside the effort to comprehend your privileges as they relate to pregnancy. In the United States, a change to Title VII of the Civil Rights Act of 1964, called The Pregnancy Discrimination Act, requires pregnant ladies to be dealt with in a way equivalent to all workers or candidates. As indicated by this demonstration, managers can't decline to contract a lady due to her pregnancy-related condition, as long as she's equipped for playing out the activity's significant capacities. If a worker is incidentally incapable to do her activity because of the pregnancy, the business must treat her equivalent to some other briefly debilitated representative, accepting such activities as giving elective undertakings, inability leave, or leave without pay. An inability may emerge because of the pregnancy itself. For example, noteworthy queasiness and spewing. A handicap may likewise happen because of difficulties of pregnancy, for example, dying, preterm work, or hypertension, or may happen because of dangerous work exposures. On the off chance that your social insurance supplier chooses that your pregnancy is crippling, you can ask that she send a letter to your boss, checking your handicap.

Health care coverage gave by a business should cover costs for pregnancy-related conditions such that it is like its inclusion of other ailments, as long as obstetric administrations are secured.

Wellbeing safety net providers are precluded by law from thinking about pregnancy as a prior condition, which implies you can't be denied inclusion when you move between various jobs and switch wellbeing plans.

# Chapter 4:
# Exercise and Dietary Requirements for A Pregnant Woman

*You will learn*

---

*Ideal bodyweight of the baby and the mother*

*Changing your diet*

*Consider food safety*

*Stay healthy when you are pregnant*

---

Through different times, women have received different advice regarding their general health and they have also been bombarded with tips regarding the food items and their overall body. This is due to the different cultural backgrounds and the latest scientific research in this field. Women were encouraged to eat a lot of food at some time and many people believed that eating a lot of food will keep the mother and baby healthy. You need to stay away from homemade tips when it comes to pregnancy and discusses your diet and exercise regime with your doctor.

Health does not always depend on eating well. You also need to do some exercise to ensure that you have healthy muscles and stay fir during your pregnancy. In this chapter, you will learn about the tips and tricks to stay in shape during your pregnancy and how to properly care for the dietary needs of your child.

## Healthy Weight Gain

It is advised that you gain weight gradually and keep your body in a fit shape if you want your baby to grow normally. Now you must be wondering about what healthy weight gain is and the issues related to weight that you might face during pregnancy. Read through this section to know more about the healthy weight and body mass.

**Understanding How Much Weight Is Good**

Body mass index is the number that is achieved by analyzing your height and weight. You need to make sure that you look at the weight gain with the help of the body mass index and discuss this with your doctor. For a normal female, a BMI of 16-22 is considered normal. This value will change for a pregnant lady. Your doctor will tell you about the healthy BMI number for a pregnant woman.

You also need to know that these numbers do not represent the actual weight gain. Gaining less weight in the early stages of the pregnancy is vital as this will also help the healthy growth of the fetus and will also make sure that the vitamins are supplied to the baby. Some women tend to put a lot of weight in the early weeks of their pregnancy and this can be unhealthy later on.

You can take help from the weight charts and use them as a guide to maintain your weight. However, these weight charts are only for your help and you should not obsess over your weight. According to the doctors, even if the mother is gaining weight abnormally, there is a strong chance that the baby's growth will be normal. Both are women who gain a lot of weight during pregnancy and those who gain very less can have healthy babies.

The doctor will use the fundal height to measure the baby's growth and ignore if your weight is off the chart. It would be alarming if you have deviated entirely from your weight class and this is the time when the doctor will probably recommend healthy food items and a strict diet.

**Knowing your infant's weight gain**

Even though your weight increase may pursue away the entirety of its own, your infant's own building up design is probably going to advance gradually from the outset, and afterward get up at around 32 weeks, just to slow again in the most recent weeks before birth. At 14 to 15 weeks, for instance, the infant puts on weight at about 0.18 ounce (5 grams) every day, and at 32 to 34 weeks, 1.06 to 1.23 ounces (30 to 35 grams) every day (that is about a large portion of a pound or 0.23 kilograms every week). Following 36 weeks, the fetal development rate eases back to about a fourth of a pound for each week, and by 41 to 42 weeks (you're past due now), negligible or no further fetal development may happen.

Notwithstanding your eating routine and weight gain, the accompanying variables influence fetal development:

Cigarette smoking: Smoking can lessen the birth weight by about a large portion of a pound (around 200 grams).

Diabetes: If the mother is diabetic, the child can be too huge or excessively little.

Genetic or family ancestry: at the end of the day, ballplayers, for the most part, don't have youngsters who grow up to be proficient racers!

Fetal disease: Some contaminations influence development, even though others don't.

Illicit medication use: Drug misuse can slow fetal development.

Mother's therapeutic history: Some restorative issues, similar to hypertension or lupus, can influence fetal development.

Multiple pregnancies: Twins and triplets are regularly littler than single children.

Placental capacity: Placental bloodstream that is worse than average can hinder the child's development.

Your expert watches out for your child's development rate, frequently by estimating fundal stature and focusing on your weight gain. On the off chance that you put on excessively little or a lot of weight, if your fundal tallness estimations are unusual, or if something in your history puts you in danger for development problems, your primary care physician is probably going to send you for an ultrasound test to more accurately survey the circumstance.

## Understanding What You Are Eating

Adhering to a well-adjusted, low-fat, high-fiber diet is significant for your child as well as for your own wellbeing. Devouring satisfactory protein is additionally significant because protein does a considerable lot of the body's capacities. The fiber in your eating routine anticipates or lessen blockage and hemorrhoids. By not devouring an excess of fat, you help keep your heart solid and abstain from putting on additional pounds that might be hard to shed. Keeping away from extreme weight gain likewise diminishes your odds of creating stretch imprints.

If your eating routine is adjusted and not very much in sugar or fat, you don't have to alter the manner in which you eat drastically. During pregnancy, you should take in about 300 additional calories daily, by and large. That implies that in case you're at a solid weight and you're taking in 2,100 calories for each day, while pregnant you should take in a normal of 2,400 calories every day (maybe somewhat less during your first trimester and somewhat more during your third trimester).

You ought not to build your caloric admission by eating a hot fudge sundae consistently. Filling these extra necessities with nutritious nourishments is critical. Your professional will probably encourage you to take some supplemental vitamins and minerals, as well. Continue perusing to discover which nourishments and enhancements are best for you.

### Utilizing the USDA Food Guide Pyramid

No single nourishment can fulfill all your wholesome needs. The USDA Food Guide Pyramid is a general rule that delineates the relative extents of servings you ought to eat in each gathering. To get some particular suggestions customized for your pre-pregnancy weight and activity level, go to www.mypyramid.gov and click on the "Pregnancy and Breastfeeding" interface.

The USDA Food Guide Pyramid incorporates the accompanying nutritional categories. They show up from left to directly on the pyramid:

Grains: Foods produced using wheat, rice, oats, cornmeal, or grain will be grain items. Entire grain nourishments contain the whole grain bit, including the wheat (the external defensive layer of the grain) and the germ (the little territory at the base of each grain). Instances of entire grains incorporate entire wheat, bulgur (broke wheat), oats, entire cornmeal, and dark colored rice. Refined grains have experienced a procedure that evacuates their wheat and germ layers, which additionally expels a great part of the fiber and a portion of the supplements, similar to B vitamins and E vitamins. Instances of refined grain items incorporate white flour, white bread, white rice, and pasta.

A normal lady needs around 6 to 8 ounces of grains for each day during pregnancy. The USDA prescribes making in any event half of your grain admission as entire grains. This implies eating around 3 to 4 ounces of entire grain bread, entire grain oat, entire grain pasta, or other entire grain items consistently.

Vegetables: Vegetables are separated into five gatherings, in view of their supplement content. The accompanying rundown orders them from most noteworthy vitamin content (dull green vegetables) to least (different vegetables), and incorporates models inside every class:

Dark green vegetables: Spinach, dull green verdant lettuce, romaine lettuce, broccoli, kale, turnip greens, watercress

Orange vegetables: Carrots; pumpkin; sweet potatoes and oak seed.

Dry beans/peas: Pinto, dark, garbanzo, kidney, naval force, soy, and white beans; split peas; lentils; tofu

Starchy vegetables: Potatoes, corn, green peas, green lima beans

Other vegetables: Cabbage, cauliflower, the chunk of ice lettuce, green beans, celery, green and red peppers, mushrooms, onions, tomatoes, asparagus, cucumbers, eggplant

Pregnant ladies should attempt to eat 21/2 to 3 cups of vegetables every day. Any of the above vegetables or unadulterated vegetable juice checks towards this objective, yet dull green or orange vegetables and dried beans are ideal since their supplement content is higher. Eating a wide range of vegetables is likewise significant, however.

Fruits: An assortment of organic products is a significant piece of your eating diet while you are pregnant. Organic products are not just a decent wellspring of vitamins and minerals; however, they likewise give fiber, which is significant during pregnancy to help diminish obstruction. Natural products contain solid measures of vitamins An and C, just as potassium.

Pregnant ladies should attempt to eat 2 to 21/2 cups of organic products every day. You can pick new, solidified, canned, or dried natural products. Go simple on the natural product juices, however, because they can contain heap added sugar.

Oils and Fats: Oils are fats that stay fluid at room temperature, similar to vegetable oil, olive oil, and corn oil. These fats are generally unsaturated and are the most advantageous sort of fats to eat. Nourishments like nuts, avocados, fish, and olives are normally high in unsaturated fats. Strong fats will be fats that are strong at room temperature, similar to margarine, shortening, grease, and blemish garine. These nourishments are high in soaked fats. Trans fats are a sort of immersed fats that are normal in prepared nourishments and have been associated with weight and coronary illness.

In a perfect world, less than 20 to 35 percent of your all-out calories should originate from fats, with less than 10 percent originating from soaked fats and trans fats being kept away from by and large.

Milk Products: Foods that fall in this gathering incorporate milk, yogurt, and cheddar, and all are incredible wellsprings of calcium. It's ideal to concentrate on low-fat or without fat milk items at whatever point conceivable. A normally measured lady needs to devour around three cups of a drain or milk items every day.

Meat and Beans: Meat, poultry, fish, dry beans, and nuts fall into this class. You should concentrate on low-fat and lean nourishments in this class and differ your decisions. Preparing, searing, and flame broiling are the most advantageous approaches to cook these nourishments. During pregnancy, you ought to eat five to seven ounces of nourishment from this classification day by day.

In case you're having this sickness and can't eat a well-adjusted eating routine, you may think whether you're getting enough sustenance that you and the baby needs. You really can go for half a month not eating an ideal eating diet with no evil impacts on the child. You may find that the main nourishments you can endure are nourishments overwhelming in starch or sugars. On the off chance that all you want to eat are potatoes, bread, and pasta, proceed. Holding something down is superior to starving.

As your pregnancy advances, your body needs a great deal of additional liquid. At an early stage, a few ladies who don't drink enough fluid feel powerless or swoon. Later in pregnancy, drying out can prompt untimely compressions. Try drinking a lot of water (or milk) — around six to eight glasses per day, and more on the off chance that you are conveying more than one infant.

**Enhancing your eating diet**

On the off chance that your eating diet is sound and adjusted, you get the greater part of the vitamins and minerals you usually need — except for iron, folic acid, and calcium. To ensure you get enough of these supplements and to guarantee against deficient dietary patterns, your expert is probably going to suggest pre-birth vitamins. On account of vitamins, more isn't really better; take just the endorsed number of pills every day. A few distinctive pre-birth vitamins are accessible, and they are commonly comparable. Some are preferred endured over others, so If you locate the one, you're taking isn't pleasing to you, attempt an alternate brand.

Additionally, many contain omega-3 unsaturated fat supplementation. A few information recommends that omega-3 enhancements may diminish the danger of pre-term conveyance and may beneficially affect the infant cerebrum, yet this hasn't been demonstrated with assurance.

If you miss taking a vitamin, don't stress. Nothing awful will occur. During the early months, if your vitamins make you sick, skipping them until you feel better is splendidly ok for the child. Keep in mind that the child is still exceptionally little, without enormous nourishing necessities. In case you're right off the bat in your pregnancy (four to seven weeks), you can take only a folic acid enhancement, which is some of the time simpler to endure until you can deal with the total pre-birth vitamin pill. If later on in the pregnancy you get a stomach infection and can't endure vitamins for quite a while, that is not an issue either. The developing child can get what it needs, even to the detriment of the mother

On the off chance that you find that the vitamins truly make you queasy, have a go at eating a couple of wafers before you take them, or take them at sleep time.

**Is caffeine safe during pregnancy?**

Albeit a few ladies believe that the main nourishment that contains caffeine is a solid mug of espresso, truth be told, you can discover caffeine in a large number of different things you eat and drink regularly: tea, numerous soft drinks, cocoa, and chocolate. No proof recommends that caffeine causes Infertility. Be that as it may, on the off chance that you expend caffeine in enormous sums, it might raise the danger of unnatural birth cycle.

Most studies propose that it takes more than 200 milligrams (mg) of caffeine daily to influence the embryo. The normal mug of espresso (remember, this is an 8-ounce cup of ordinary espresso — not the supersize or a coffee or top cappuccino!) has somewhere in the range of 100 and 150 mg of caffeine. Energized tea has somewhat less caffeine — around 50 to 100 mg — and soda pops have roughly 36 mg for each 12-ounce serving. So, drinking one 8-ounce mug of espresso (or the proportionate caffeine content in different nourishments or refreshments) every day is typically alright during pregnancy. Plenty of ladies get some information about the caffeine content in chocolate — your sweet tooth will be glad to realize that a normal estimated chocolate bar or a cup of hot cocoa has just around 6 mg of caffeine.

Keep in mind that expending caffeine regularly expands the effectively visit outings to the washroom. In case you're as of now pestered by visit pee, you might need to cut your caffeine consumption further. Additionally, you may find that, particularly in the last trimester, getting an entire night's rest is practically outlandish because you can't discover a solace capable dozing position and, regardless of whether you do, you need to get up a few times to go to the restroom. Drinking espresso or tea in the evening may just exasperate your failure to get some rest!

**Iron**

You need increasingly iron when you're expecting because both you and the infant are making new red platelets consistently. All things considered, you need 30 milligrams (mg) of additional iron each day of your pregnancy, which is the thing that most pre-birth vitamins contain. Blood tallies can without much of a stretch drop during pregnancy because your body step by step is making increasingly more blood plasma (liquid) and moderately fewer red platelets (which is known as dilutional frailty). On the off chance that you do create sickliness, you may need to take an additional iron enhancement.

Nourishments wealthy in iron incorporate chicken, fish, red meat, verdant green vegetables, and enhanced or bread and oats. You can raise the iron substance of nourishments by cooking them in cast-iron pots and skillets.

**Calcium and vitamin D**

You need around 1,200 milligrams of calcium and 2,000 units of Vitamin D consistently while you're pregnant. (The U.S. Suggested Daily Allowance [USRDA] of calcium for all ladies is around 1,000 mg.) Most ladies really get considerably less. In case you're now beginning to some degree calcium and vitamin D insufficient, the calcium prerequisites of the creating infant will just exacerbate the situation for you. A baby can remove enough calcium from its mom, regardless of whether it implies getting it to the detriment of the mother's bones. So, the additional calcium and vitamin D required during pregnancy are truly planned for ensuring you and your wellbeing. Vitamin D causes you to store the calcium.

Pre-birth vitamins contain just around 200 to 300 mg of calcium (around one-fourth of the USRDA), so you have to get calcium from different sources also.

Getting enough calcium from your eating diet alone is conceivable on the off chance that you truly focus. You can get it from three to four servings of calcium-rich nourishments, for example, milk, yogurt, cheddar, verdant green vegetables, and canned fish with bones (if your stomach can take it). General stores likewise stock exceptional without lactose nourishments that are high in calcium.

## Knowing Which Food Items Are Safe

At the point when our patients get some information about sustenance and which nourishments they might need to keep away from, specific things come up over and over. This segment distinguishes the possibly unsafe nourishments and furthermore shed light on some normal legends about different food sources.

**Some harmful nourishments to look out for**

When you are healthy you can presumably eat the greater part of the nourishments your partner eats. In any case, the accompanying rundown contains some potential perils that we believe we should specify:

Cheeses from unpasteurized or crude milk: Cheeses produced using unpasteurized or ballplayers' milk may contain certain microbes, for example, listeria, monocytogenes, salmonella, and E. coli. Listeria, specifically, has been connected to certain pregnancy intricacies, for example, untimely work or even premature delivery. The FDA commands that all cheeses sold in the United States be either produced using purified milk or matured over 60 days (which makes the probability of listeria very low), so most cheeses you purchase at your neighborhood advertise are protected. Simply check the name no doubt.

Raw or exceptionally uncommon meat: Steak tartare or extremely uncommon hamburger or pork may contain microorganisms, for example, listeria, or parasites, for example, toxoplasma. Sufficient cooking slaughters the two microorganisms and parasites. At the end of the day, you need your nourishment to be cooked medium-well to very much done.

Liver: Because it contains amazingly high measures of Vitamin An (more than the sum prescribed for a pregnant lady), liver devoured in early pregnancy may speculatively be connected to birth surrenders. Expending more than 10,000 global units (IUs) of Vitamin A day by day (the suggested day by day remittance for pregnant ladies is 2,500 IU) was connected to birth absconds in one examination. Researchers haven't demonstrated this risk unequivocally, yet you might need to locate a substitute for that liver and onions desiring in the main trimester. Also, look at the name on your pre-birth vitamins to ensure you're not getting a lot of Vitamin A.

**Popular Food Myths to Know About**

The food items that have once or twice harmed a pregnant woman is unlikely to harm you as well. You need to make sure that you take special care when you are eating these food items as they can cause problems when you are pregnant.

Aspartame (Equal or Nutrasweet): Aspartame (a typical part of low-calorie nourishments and refreshments) is a kind of amino acid, and the body is acquainted with amino acids since they're what all proteins are made of. No therapeutic proof shows that aspartame brings on any issues for the developing infant.

Sucralose (Splenda): Sucralose is one of the freshest low-calorie available, with under 2 calories for each teaspoon. It is really a kind of sugar, however, it's substantially more powerful than customary table sugar, so you just need modest quantities to improve things up (and in this way you get fewer calories). Since it's a sort of sugar, it should have no unsafe consequences for your creating infant.

Cheeses: Not just do the vast majority accept that prepared and pasteurized cheeses are sheltered, yet these cheeses are additionally an incredible wellspring of both protein and calcium. See the segment "Looking at possibly destructive nourishments" for data about unpasteurized cheeses.

Fish: Fish is an extraordinary wellspring of protein and vitamins, and is additionally low in fat. Truth be told, the significant levels of protein, omega-3 unsaturated fats, vitamin D, and different supplements make fish amazing nourishment for pregnant moms and their creating babies. Be that as it may, certain fish — shark, mackerel, swordfish, and tilefish — contain elevated levels of mercury. The jury's still out on whether mercury may prompt certain youth formative postponements or issues with fine engine abilities (presumably not), however, the FDA as of now suggests you keep away from fish with elevated levels of mercury when you're pregnant.

The USDA rules state you can, in any case, appreciate up to 12 ounces (2 normal dinners) every seven-day stretch of fish and shellfish lower in mercury, similar to salmon, tilapia, cod, sole, and shrimp or up to 6 ounces of tuna fish every week. (The restrictions are because of the way that even fish that is low in mercury isn't sans mercury, so mercury utilization could mean a significant sum if fish were eaten in huge amounts.) Don't give your anxiety for mercury a chance to make you surrender fish by and large since two late investigations taking a gander at fish utilization in pregnant ladies indicated that ladies who eat fish may really have lower paces of preterm conveyance, and their children may have higher IQs than the individuals who don't eat fish.

Sushi: Raw fish (with the exception of crude shellfish) really conveys an extremely little danger of parasitic contamination (around one disease in 2,000,000 servings), regardless of whether you're pregnant or not (this is not exactly the danger of becoming ill from eating chicken!). Pregnancy doesn't build the risk, and your hatchling is probably not going to experience the ill effects of such contamination. Most significant is to ensure that the fish originates from a dependable source and that it is put away appropriately.

Smoked meats or fish: Many pregnant ladies stress overeating smoked meats and fish since they've heard that these nourishments are high in nitrites or nitrates. In spite of the fact that these nourishments do contain these substances, they won't hurt your child whenever eaten with some restraint.

## Considering Special Dietary Needs

When you try to follow the strict dietary regime provided by the doctor, you will have a fair problem related to digestion., for example, obstruction or acid reflux. Or on the other hand, you may find that you have to tailor the guidelines to accommodate your specific dietary patterns — for instance, in case you're a vegan. In this area, we address a portion of the issues that emerge for ladies with extraordinary dietary contemplations and for all ladies who may encounter any stomach related issues.

## Eating right, veggie lover style

In case you're a veggie-lover, have confidence that you can deliver a solid infant without eating steak. In any case, you do need to design your eating routine all the more cautiously. Vegetables, entire grains, and vegetables (peas and beans) are wealthy in protein, yet most don't have total proteins. (They don't contain all the basic amino acids that your body can't deliver without anyone else's input.) To get all the vital protein, you can join different proteins, for instance, entire grains with vegetables or nuts, rice with kidney beans, or even nutty spread with entire grain bread. The blend doesn't need to happen at a similar supper, just around the same time, however, a decent dependable guideline is to attempt to get some protein with every feast.

If you don't eat any creature items, including drain and cheddar, your eating routine may not give enough of six other significant supplements: vitamin B12, calcium, riboflavin, iron, zinc, and vitamin D. Raise the subject with your primary care physician. You may likewise need to talk about your eating routine with a nutritionist.

**Fighting Constipation**

Progesterone, a hormone that courses openly through your body during pregnancy, can hinder your stomach related framework and subsequently cause stoppage. The additional iron from your pre-birth vitamin just exacerbates the situation. Ladies who are on bed rest in light of pregnancy difficulties are at specific danger of obstruction since they're so inert.

You can balance blockage by drinking a lot of liquids, by eating satisfactory fiber (as organic products, vegetables, beans, wheat, and other entire grains), and, if conceivable, by getting exercise each day. Remember, be that as it may, that a few ladies experience stomach uneasiness, swelling, or gas from eating a lot of nourishments high in fiber. You may need to utilize a little experimentation to see which fiber-rich nourishments you endure best. If obstruction disturbs you, your expert may suggest a stool conditioner.

**Managing diabetes**

In case you have diabetes or you get diabetes during pregnancy, change your eating routine with the goal that it incorporates explicit amounts of proteins, fats, and starches to guarantee that you keep up a typical degree of blood glucose (sugar).

Incredible wellness development hasn't left pregnant ladies behind. You see them running in parks, turning out in exercise centers, or extending their appendages in yoga classes. During pregnancy, exercise helps your body from multiple points of view: It keeps your heart solid and your muscles fit as a fiddle, and it eases the essential stress of pregnancy — from morning affliction to obstruction to pain-filled legs and backs. In the 40 weeks a pregnant woman needs to exercise her body to make her keep fit. So, in case, you're healthy and not in danger for obstetrical or medicinal complexities, by all methods feel free to proceed with your activity program — except if your program calls for climbing Mount Fuji, entering an expert bout, or some different super strenuous movement. Go over your activity program with your professional, so he can advise.

## Adjusting to Your Body's Progressions

Regardless of whether you turn out with some restraint, recall that pregnancy makes your body experience genuine physical changes that can influence your quality, stamina, and execution. The accompanying rundown subtletles a portion of those changes:

Cardiovascular changes: When you're pregnant, the measure of blood that your heart siphons through your body increments. That expansion in blood volume, as a rule, has no impact on your exercise. (A few ladies can feel as if they hear their pulse in their ears as a result of the expanded volume.) Also, if you lie level on your back, particularly after around about four months of pregnancy, you may wind up feeling unsteady or swoon — or even queasy. Known as recumbent hypotension disorder, this wooziness some of the time happens when the expanding uterus pushes down on significant veins that arrival blood to the heart, along these lines diminishing the heart's yield. It hap-pens significantly more promptly in case you're conveying a various pregnancy and your uterus is that a lot heavier.

In case you're doing any activities that expect you to lie on your back (or in case you're acquainted with dozing on your back), put a little cushion or froth wedge under the correct side of your back or your correct hip. The pad tilts you marginally sideways and adequately lift your uterus off the veins.

Respiratory changes: Your body is utilizing more oxygen than expected to help the developing infant. Simultaneously, breathing is more work than it used to be because the extending uterus presses upward against the stomach. For certain ladies, this trouble makes performing oxygen consuming activity somewhat harder.

Structural changes: As your body shape changes — greater guts, bigger bosoms — your focal point of gravity shifts, which can influence your equalization. The weight shift can be felt when you are walking or driving a bike or a ski. We recommend that you limit your movement when you are deep into pregnancy. What's more, pregnancy hormones cause some remissness in your joints, which likewise can make balance increasingly troublesome and may build your danger of damage.

Metabolic changes: Pregnant ladies use starches quicker than nonpregnant ladies do, which implies that they're at a higher danger of creating hypoglycemia (low glucose). Exercise can be valuable in helping lower and control glucose levels; however, it additionally builds the body's requirement for sugars. So, if you work out, ensure that you're eating a sufficient measure of starch just before you work out.

Effects on the uterus: One investigation of ladies at term (far enough along to convey) indicated that their constrictions expanded after moderate oxygen consuming activity. Another study demonstrated that activity is related to a lower danger of early work. Be that as it may, most investigations have demonstrated that activity has no impact in any case, and exercise doesn't represent a danger of preterm work in solid pregnant ladies.

Effect on birth weight: Some examinations have demonstrated that ladies who work out strenuously (at high power) during pregnancy have lighter-weight babies. A similar impact seems to happen in ladies who perform overwhelming physical work in a standing position while they're pregnant. the reduction in the baby weight is mostly caused due to less fat in the baby and there is no effect of exercise on the baby health.

**Excersing Without Trying Too Hard**

Your changing body is going to request a changing activity schedule. Try not to pound yourself If you find that pregnancy makes it harder to proceed with the exercises you're acclimated with. Alter your program as per what you can sensibly endure.

Tune in to your body. On the off chance that weightlifting all of a sudden damage your back, help up. You may think that it is simpler to perform no weight-bearing activities like swimming or stationary bicycling. Regardless of what your specific practice routine might be, remember the fundamental rules for working out during pregnancy:

If you have a moderate exercise schedule, keep it up. If you've been inactive, don't abruptly dive into a strenuous program; ease in gradually to abstain from putting an excessive amount of strain on your body. Keep in mind that keeping up a normal calendar of moderate action is superior to taking part in inconsistent spurts of exceptional exercise, which are bound to cause damage.

Avoid practicing level on your back for significant periods; doing so may lessen bloodstream to your heart.

Try not to overheat or get got dried out, and if you feel exhausted, bleary-eyed, blackout, or queasy, by all methods stop. On hot or moist days, don't practice outside.

Avoid whatever puts you in danger of being harmed in the midriff, similar to street/mountain biking.

Steer clear of high-sway, fun activities that can assess your relaxing joints.

Throughout the nine months, low-or moderate-sway exercises bode well than high-sway ones.

Carry a jug of water to each activity session and remain all around hydrated.

Eat a well-adjusted eating diet that incorporates a sufficient inventory of starches (see "Considering What You're Taking In," before this section).

Talk to your specialist about what your pinnacle practice pulse ought to be. (Numerous professionals recommend 140 pulsates every moment as far as possible.) Then consistently measure your pulse at the pinnacle of your exercise to ensure that it's at a protected level. Whenever you feel the shortness of breath or dizziness, you need to stop working and contact your doctor. Rapid heartbeat is another cause of concern for the pregnant women and consultation with a gynecologist is recommended when you feel it.

**Diverse pregnant women exercises**

When you are pregnant, you need to take a proper diet and avoid heavy exercise. Aiming for the bikini body when you are pregnant can be dangerous for you and your child. So, exercise carefully and it is advised that you work under the professional fitness instructor as they will help you keep a fit body without harming your health.

You can do the walking, running and different types of aerobic exercises without any issue. Never work out for more than an hour when you are pregnant. The shift in the center of gravity and the weight of the baby will make it difficult to exercise. If possible, limit the exercise otherwise you can harm the baby. Always do the exercise in which you are comfortable and do not attempt new things, as you do not want to do anything that can harm your body or your baby.

Apart from the aerobic exercises, you can also do the Pilates that is a mind and body fitness program that is focused on core postural muscles. When you do pilates, give your body some time to heal. You need to look for specialized courses for pregnant women when you are planning to work out.

Weight-less and bodyweight exercises are best for pregnant women. As you will not have to work with wright and your weight will be supported, there is a small chance of any injury. You will put less stress on your joints. If you are new to the exercise, it is advised that you start off with low-intensity workouts.

Some activities such as downhill skiing and horseback riding are prohibited by the doctors during pregnancy.

# Chapter 5:
# The First Trimester

*You will learn*

---

*The body changes in early pregnancy*

*Baby's development in the first twelve week*

*Knowing concerns and issues of pregnancy*

*Involving your partner*

---

Being pregnant for the first time is quite tantalizing and alluring. You feel a lot of body changes and experience things that you have not felt before. The infant goes through a lot of changes in the first 12 weeks. The baby will start to grow organs in this time. Fatigue be one of the major concerns for you in the first trimester. You will also develop tender breasts. Seeing a medical officer in the first trimester is important and he/she will surely guide you on how to make this process easy for you.

## A New Life Begins

You may know by now that pregnancy begins when the sperm meets the egg and this process is completed in the fallopian tube. When sperm and egg meet, they form a single cell called zygote. The zygote will divide many times and will form a blastocyst and it will travel to the uterus. When the blastocyst reaches the womb, you will start feeling many changes in your body. Implantation – the process in which the blastocyst attaches to the lining to uterus usually happens after five days of its development.

Some parts of the blastocyst will grow to become the placenta and the other will form the embryo. The embryo will be called a fetus after eight weeks of its development. By this time, all the major organs of the baby will be formed. In eight weeks, the toes, arms, legs, and fingers of the baby will be formed. You will also start to feel and see the little movements of the embryo after eight weeks and they will also be clear during the first ultrasound. In 12 weeks, the fetus will be around 1 ounce and will be 4 inches long.

## Know that body changes you should expect in pregnancy

You need to prepare yourself for major changes in the body. The baby inside you will grow and your body will adjust to it. These adjustments will not be as comfortable as you think. Read along to know the changes in the first twelve weeks.

# EARLY PREGNANCY

- Placenta
- Uterus
- Cervix
- Vagina
- Amniotic Fluid
- Amnion
- Chorion

*Double arrow indicates crown-rumplength

**MOMMY'S ANGELS**
EDITORIAL STAFF
GROW YOUR TODDLER TO THE BEST!

**Changes in the Breast**

Changes in the breast are probably the first thing that you will notice in your body. During the first month, the breasts will feel more tender and will start to grow. The nipples and the areolae will darken and being to grow. Estrogen increase causes these breast changes. These changes and rise in estrogen are due to the anticipation of breastfeeding after the baby is born. You will also notice that the blood supply to the breast will increase. Be prepared to purchase new bras when pregnant. Women might feel self-conscious when their breast has grown but this is a natural process and you should not be embarrassed about it.

**Fatigue**

Be prepared to feel tired all the time. It is caused due to body changes. The rise in the hormones and the fatigue is likely to go away by 12 to 14 weeks after your pregnancy. This fatigue is like a signal that your body is giving. Doctors suggest that you take more rest when you are pregnant. This fatigue will go away after 12 weeks and you will feel almost normal.

**Sickness During the Day**

You will feel nauseated during the first trimester and you will feel its full effect in the morning when you have an empty stomach. The morning sickness lasts until 12 weeks of the pregnancy and this condition may last longer in women who are expecting twins or triplets.

You should understand nausea during pregnancy is inevitable so instead of finding ways to cure it, you need to consult with a doctor and learn the precautionary measures that you should take. You need to contact your doctor when you are losing weight rapidly and feeling dizzy all the time.

**Bloating**

Your belly will become bloated before the child can stretch your tummy and begin to take shape. This may be uncomfortable at first but you will get used to it as time passes. When you conceive, the production of the hormone in the body will change and progesterone – the production of the hormone responsible for retaining water will increase. Belly size is also increased due to estrogen. It will retain the bowels and cause them to enlarge. Uterus size will also increase due to the increase of estrogen. You will feel increased bloating in the second and third trimester.

**Urination Issues**

Increased urination is another problem that you have to face. You will have to urinate a lot during pregnancy. When you are pregnant, the size of the bladder decreases that results in storing less urine. It is recommended that you urinate before you travel or visit any place. The urination during the pregnancy is inevitable and with common sense and a healthy diet, you can decrease the frequency of urination. There is an increased chance of urinary tract infection during pregnancy so you need to take caution when you are pregnant. Contact the doctor when you feel blood in the urine.

**Headaches**

Most women feel increased headaches during pregnancy. The headaches may be caused due to the sudden decrease in the blood pressure, fatigue, nausea or bouts of hunger. Many doctors recommend the simple dose of ibuprofen or Advil when you are suffering from headaches. Many women have relief from a single cup of coffee and some use the combination of different medicines to tackle the headache. The doctor will check your symptoms and will prescribe a mild tranquilizer if over-the-counter medications do not work properly.

## Constipation

Pregnant women need to face constipation regularly. According to the reports, more than 50 percent women reportedly faced this issue during the first 12 weeks. Progesterone increase in the body causes constipation. Most pregnant women use iron supplements that also cause constipation. Follow these simple suggestions to deal with constipation:

**Use high-fiber food items:** Increase the fiber intake and use food items such as vegetables, fruits, and cereals to get rid of digestion problems. You should choose food items with high fiber content.

**Increase your water intake:** Increasing your water intake will help you to move the food and waste within your digestive system. Apple and prune juice may also help to reduce constipation.

**Exercise Regularly:** This will surely help you to eliminate constipation from your life when you are pregnant.

**Use Stool Softeners:** Products such as Docusate Sodium will help in keeping the stool soft. The stool softener can be used during pregnancy Use the stool softener 3 to 4 times a day.

## The First Prenatal Appointment

On the first prenatal appointment, the doctor will share facts regarding pregnancy; the prenatal visits during pregnancy are frequent and important. These checkups ensure the health of your baby. You should also bring the father-to-be in the prenatal visits as checking his family background and ethnic roots are also important. This will be the best chance for the father to voice his concerns and find out what he should expect in the next months.

The doctors will have many things to discuss and need to make different checkup and this is why; it may take more than an hour. The next visits will be shorter – such as 10-15 minutes. The frequency of prenatal visits depends upon your medical condition and complications. A medical officer recommends one visit every four weeks. The baby's heartbeat, your urine and body will be checked in this session.

**Lifestyle**

How a person lives and works may affect childbirth and pregnancy. The doctor will inquire about your lifestyle and will ask about your job requirement; for example, if you have to lift heavy objects on the job or you have a sedentary job. The doctor will also inquire about your exercise patterns, diet restriction, and smoking.

**The last menstrual period**

Remember the date of the last period and this will help in determining the due date. If you do not even remember the conceiving date, the doctor will do an ultrasound to know how far along you are.

**Gynecological History**

If you have not scheduled a preconception visit, the doctor will surely ask you about the gynecological history. He/she will probably ask about the earlier pregnancies and problems you might have faced. Understanding your gynecological history will let them decide how to handle your pregnancy. Knowing the complete medical history gives the doctor the confidence to handle your case.

**Infertility treatment**

When you have used the infertility treatments to conceive, you should tell this to the doctor. Many complications need to be addressed when you conceive of this method. There is a chance of multi-fetal pregnancies and the doctors will prescribe the medicine according to your condition.

**Medical Problems**

Medical officer inquiries about your medical conditions and any surgeries. Many medical conditions affect the pregnancy and there are some that do not; so, share all the information with the doctor. You should also tell the doctor about the allergies that you have. The doctor needs to understand your body condition so that a healthy child is born.

**Family Medical History**

The family restorative accounts of both you and the child's dad are significant for two reasons. To start with, your professional can distinguish pregnancy-related conditions that can repeat from age to age, such as having twins or uncommonly enormous infants. The other explanation is to recognize significant issues inside your family that your infant can acquire. Blood tests can screen for a portion of these issues, for example, cystic fibrosis. If there is a family ancestry of mental impediment or learning incapacities, examine the choice for Fragile X disorder screening with your primary care physician or hereditary advisor. Delicate X disorder is the most well-known acquired reason for mental impediment and results from a variation from the norm in the X chromosome. The pre-birth analysis is accessible for Fragile X disorder if your family ancestry recommends this plausibility.

**Ethnic roots**

Studying the ethnic roots can help the doctor to know about any concerning points. Jewish individuals of Eastern European drop, for instance, are multiple times more probable than others to convey the uncommon quality for Tay-Sachs, an ailment of the sensory system that is generally lethal in early adolescence. French Canadians and Cajuns (from Louisiana) likewise have a higher-than-ordinary danger of conveying this quality.

More often than not, a straightforward blood test can decide if you're a transporter of this infection. Another ethnically specific ailment is sickle-cell pallor, a blood issue that is particularly common among individuals with African or Hispanic progenitors. This condition, as well, is latent, so the two individuals from a couple must be transporters for the infant to be in danger of acquiring the ailment.

Individuals whose progenitors originate from Italy, Greece, and other Mediterranean nations are at raised danger of having — and going to their youngsters — qualities for the blood issue beta-thalassemia, otherwise called Mediterranean pallor or Cooley's iron deficiency. Among Asians, the undifferentiated from blood issue is alpha-thalassemia. Both of these disarranges produce variations from the norm in hemoglobin (the protein in red platelets that clutches oxygen) and thusly bring about differing degrees of pallor. Like Tay-Sachs and sickle-cell iron deficiency, the two guardians need to convey the quality all together for their child to be in danger of having the illness.

**Screening for cystic fibrosis**

CF is additionally a passive condition, similar to Tay-Sachs (see the "Ethnic roots" segment). More than 1,250 distinctive hereditary changes have been related to CF. As of now, obstetricians and geneticists prescribe that CF screening be offered to every pregnant couple. Since the possibility of being a bearer is more noteworthy in the Ashkenazi Jewish and Caucasian populaces, screening (by a blood test) ought to be performed if at any rate one partner is Jewish or Caucasian. Screening for the 23 most basic transformations will get 57 to 97 percent of transporters of cystic fibrosis, contingent upon the ethnic foundation. (For instance, it distinguishes 97 percent of bearers among the Ashkenazi Jewish populace, 80 percent of transporters in the Northern European Caucasian populace, and 57 percent of transporters in the American Hispanic populace.) Speak to your primary care physician about CF screening during your first pre-birth visit.

The dangers of inheritable infections cover starting with one ethnic or geographic gathering then onto the next. Qualities get went around among the different populaces at whatever point the guardians are from various ethnic gatherings. In any case, you can generally measure whether your parentage puts you at a raised danger of conveying qualities for specific ailments.

A few people don't know particularly about their ethnic foundation or family restorative history, maybe because they were received or haven't had a lot of contact with their organic families. If this circumstance is valid for your situation, don't stress. Remember that the odds that both you and your partner convey a quality for a specific issue are very low.

**Thinking about the physical test**

At your first pre-birth visit, your professional analyzes your head, neck, bosoms, heart, lungs, belly, and limits. She likewise plays out an interior test. During this test, your specialist assesses your uterus, cervix, and ovaries, and performs, if due, a PAP test (cervix malignancy and pre-disease screening). If you believe you likewise ought to be tried for the probability of explicitly transmitted maladies, educate your doctor because the PAP test doesn't screen for every one of them.

After the test, you and your expert will examine the general arrangement for your pregnancy and discussion about any potential issues. You can likewise examine what drugs you can take while you're pregnant when you should call for help, and what tests you can hope to experience all through your pregnancy.

**Looking at the standard tests**

Prepare yourself: You're presumably going to be acquainted with a needle and need to pee in a cup during your first pre-birth visit. Here's a glance at the standard strategies, including blood and pee tests.

**Prepare for the prick: Blood tests**

On your first pre-birth visit, your expert will draw your blood for a lot of standard tests to check your general wellbeing, just to ensure you are safe to specific diseases. The accompanying tests are standard:

✓ A standard test for blood classification, Rh factor, and immune response status. The blood classification alludes to whether your blood is type A, B, AB, or O and whether you're Rh-positive or Rh-negative. The neutralizer test is intended to advise whether exceptional blood-bunch antibodies to specific antigens (like the Rh antigen) are available.

✓ Complete blood tally (CBC). This test checks for frailty, which alludes to a low blood tally.

✓ VDRL or RPR. These tests check for syphilis, an explicitly transmitted infection. They're precise, yet once in a while, they produce a bogus positive outcome if the patient has different conditions, for example, lupus or the antiphospholipid neutralizer disorder. Nonetheless, these sorts of bogus positive outcomes are generally feebly positive. These tests are vague, so as to affirm the conclusion of syphilis, another, increasingly explicit blood test ought to be performed. Since its fundamental that syphilis is treated, ensure you get a test. Indeed, most states require it. Tragically, the rate of syphilis is on the ascent in the United States.

✓ Hepatitis B. This test checks for proof of hepatitis infections. These infections come in a few distinct sorts, and the hepatitis B infection is one that can be available without creating genuine indications. A few ladies are analyzed distinctly during a blood test.

✓ Rubella. Your professional additionally checks for insusceptibility to rubella (likewise called German measles). Most ladies have been inoculated against rubella or, because they have had the ailment previously, their blood conveys antibodies, which is the reason the danger of contracting German measles during pregnancy is so uncommon. Most specialists test to see that the mother is invulnerable to rubella during the absolute first pre-birth visit. An expert additionally encourages these ladies to get inoculated against rubella not long after they convey, so they aren't powerless in resulting pregnancies.

✓ HIV. Since medicine is accessible to diminish the danger of transmission to the child, just as to slow sickness movement in the mother, monitoring your HIV status is significant. A specialist can generally play out this test simultaneously as the other pre-birth blood tests.

## Ultrasound in the first trimester

Ultrasound utilizes sound waves to make an image of the uterus and the infant inside it. Ultrasound assessments don't include radiation, and the technique is safe for both you and your infant. Your specialist may propose that you experience a first-trimester ultrasound test. Regularly, this ultrasound is performed transvaginal, which implies that an exceptional ultrasound test is embedded into the vagina. The favorable position to this method is that the test, or transducer, is nearer to the hatchling, so a much clearer view is achieved with a standard transabdominal ultrasound assessment. A few ladies stress that a transvaginal test embedded into the vagina could hurt the child.

**Coming up next are assessed during a first-trimester ultrasound test:**

✓       The precision of your due date: Finding the time of the last menstrual period and a simple ultrasound test will help doctors find the right due date. The ultrasound test will show the size of the baby and the doctor may change the due date according to the reports. An ultrasound in the principal trimester is, in reality, more precise than a later ultrasound in affirming or setting up your due date.

✓       Fetal reasonability: The probability of miscarriage drops to less than 3 percent when the ultrasound test is conducted to check the heartbeat of the child. Preceding five weeks, the hatchling itself may not be unmistakable; rather, the ultrasound may show just the gestational sac.

✓       Fetal anomalies: Although a total ultrasound assessment to distinguish basic variations from the norm in the hatchling ordinarily isn't performed until around 20 weeks, a few issues may as of now be unmistakable by 11 to 12 weeks. A significant part of the mind, spine, appendages, stomach area and urinary tract structures might be seen with transvaginal ultrasound. Moreover, the nearness of a thickening behind the neck of the embryo (known as expanded nuchal translucency) may show an additional hazard for certain hereditary or chromosomal conditions.

✓       Fetal number: An ultrasound shows whether you're conveying more than one baby. Furthermore, the presence of the film isolating the children, just as the placental areas, shows whether the children share one placenta or have separate placentas. We expound on this point in Chapter 15.

✓ The state of your ovaries: An ultrasound can uncover irregularities or growths in your ovaries. In some cases, an ultrasound shows a little sore, called a corpus luteal pimple. This is a blister that structures at the site where the egg was discharged. Through the span of three or four months, it continuously leaves. Two different kinds of blisters called dermoid growths and straightforward sores, are inconsequential to the pregnancy and might be found during an ultrasound test. Regardless of whether the expulsion of these sorts of growths is important and when they ought to be evacuated relies upon the size of the blister and any side affects you might be having.

✓ The nearness of fibroid tumors: Also called fibroids, these are generous abundances of the muscle of the uterus.

✓ Location of the pregnancy: Occasionally, the pregnancy might be situated outside the uterus, which is called an ectopic pregnancy.

## Perceiving Causes for Concern

In every trimester, a couple of things may go not exactly easy. The accompanying segments portray a portion of the things that can occur during the main trimester of your pregnancy and what they may intend to you.

### Bleeding

Right off the bat in pregnancy, around the hour of your missed period, encountering a touch of seeping from the vagina isn't exceptional. The measure of draining is typically not as much as what you would expect with a period and goes on for just a couple of days. This is known as implantation bleeding, and it happens when the prepared egg appends to the uterus' covering. Seeping because of implantation isn't a reason for concern, yet numerous ladies might be befuddled by it and mix-up it for their period.

Draining additionally may happen later in the main trimester, however, it doesn't really show unsuccessful labor. Around 33% of ladies experience seeping during the main trimester, and most of them proceed to have alive and well infants. Draining is particularly basic in ladies conveying more than one embryo — and once more, most proceed to have ordinary pregnancies. Splendid red draining, for the most part, demonstrates dynamic bleeding, while dim recoloring, as a rule, shows old blood that is advancing out from the cervix and vagina. You need to know that the ultrasound will not tell you if the child is dying. The main cause of the bleeding may be the seeping from the placenta. During this time, some dim blood keeps on dropping through the cervix and vagina.

This is the main hint of the unnatural birth cycle. For this situation, draining frequently goes with stomach cramping. Notwithstanding, remember that by far most of the ladies who experience draining proceed to have a totally typical pregnancy.

If you see some bleeding, let your medical expert know. In case you're draining intensely (substantially more than a period), call your specialist when you can. He or she might need to do an ultrasound and play out a pelvic test to find out the reason for the draining and see whether the pregnancy is as yet practical and situated inside the uterus. In most cases, there is no clear remedy for the bleeding. A few specialists may propose that you rest at home for a couple of days and keep away from exercise and sex. No logical information underpins these directions, however, given that no great choices exist, they surely don't hurt.

**Miscarriage**

The larger part of pregnancies continues regularly. About a fraction of the time, chromosomal variations from the norm in the developing life cause the unnatural birth cycle. In another 20 percent of cases, the developing life may have auxiliary imperfections that are too little to be in any way discernible by ultrasound or neurotic assessment. Note: Having one unsuccessful labor doesn't mean that you have an expanded possibility of it happening once more. Likewise, no schedule each day exercises can cause unsuccessful labor.

Premature delivery may be prompt by cramping and bleeding. You may feel stomach troubles that are more grounded than menstrual spasms, and you may pass fetal and placental tissue. In situations where all the tissue is passed, your medical professional doesn't have to do anything else. Frequently, however, some tissue stays in your uterus, and you may require a prescription to urge its passing or to have a D&C (dilation and curettage) method, intended to discharge the uterus. A D&C can be performed either in the specialist's office or in a labor room, contingent upon the specialist, the gestational age, and some other significant medicinal issues.

Now and then, you may have no plain indications of unsuccessful labor. Contingent upon your obstetrical history and your longing to attempt to decide the reason for the unsuccessful labor, you may choose to have the tissue sent for hereditary examination (to see if the chromosomes were ordinary or unusual). Shockingly, most unnatural birth cycles can't be anticipated. Many, if not most, of them, may basically be nature's method for taking care of an unusual pregnancy.

Nonetheless, having a premature delivery doesn't imply that you can't have a superbly typical pregnancy later on. Truth be told, even in ladies who have had two consecutive premature deliveries, the odds are excellent (around 70 percent) that the following pregnancy will be effective with no unique treatment.

Any lady who encounters a few backs to back unsuccessful labors may have a hidden condition that can be recognized and potentially treated. She ought to have a total physical assessment and experience extraordinary tests to search for causes. A few ladies who have even one unsuccessful labor might need to be inspected. If you prematurely deliver, talk about with your expert the plausibility of experiencing certain tests or sending fetal or placental tissue to a research facility for chromosomal examination.

**Ectopic pregnancy**

An ectopic pregnancy happens when the fertilized egg develops outside the uterus — in one of the fallopian tubes, the ovary, the stomach area, or the cervix. An ectopic pregnancy is a genuine risk to the mother's wellbeing. Luckily, ultrasound has progressed to the point that it can identify ectopic pregnancies early.

Indications of an ectopic pregnancy that you may see incorporate vaginal dying, stomach issues, unsteadiness, and feeling faint. The doctor will be able to find the issue with the help of ultrasound. There are different methods to treat ectopic pregnancy and the procedures depend on how much long you have been pregnant for.

# Chapter 6:
# The Second Trimester

*You will learn*

---

### LEARN THE BABY'S DEVELOPMENT

### FEELING THAT YOU ARE GOING TO BE A MOTHER

### KNOW THE CONCERNING POINTS OF THE DELIVERY

---

The sentiments of sickness and weariness so regular during the first trimester are normally gone, and you feel increasingly lively and agreeable. The subsequent trimester is an extremely energizing time since you can feel the child moving inside you and you're at last beginning to appear. During the subsequent trimester, blood tests, pre-birth tests, and ultrasound (sonogram) can affirm that the child is solid and developing typically. Furthermore, numerous ladies discover they can at long last handle the idea that they'll before long be having a child. The subsequent trimester is regularly the time you start offering the energizing news to family, companions, and collaborators.

## Finding How Your Baby Is Developing

Your child develops quickly during the subsequent trimester. The baby measures around 3 inches (8 centimeters) in length at 13 weeks. By 26 weeks, it's around 14 inches (35 centimeters) and weighs around 2 1/4 pounds (1,022 grams). Somewhere close to weeks 14 and 16, the appendages start to prolong and begin to look like arms and legs. Facilitated arm and leg developments are discernible on ultrasound, as well. The fetal developments may start in the eighteenth week. In the start, the baby's head may seem a little big for its body but as the body grows, the head becomes proportionate.

BABY GROWTH IN MOM

The bones set and are unmistakable on ultrasound. Right off the bat in the subsequent trimester, the hatchling looks something like an outsider (think E.T.), yet by 26 weeks, it looks substantially more like a human child.

The baby additionally performs numerous conspicuous exercises. It moves, yet in addition experiences normal times of resting and attentiveness and can hear and swallow. Lung advancement increments extraordinarily somewhere in the range of 20 and 25 weeks.

By 24 weeks, lung cells start to discharge surfactant, a synthetic substance that empowers the lungs to remain extended. Somewhere in the range of 26 and 28 weeks, the eyes — which had been melded closed — open, and hair (called lanugo) shows up on the head and body. Fat stores structure under the skin and the focal sensory system develops significantly.

At 23 to 24 weeks, the hatchling is viewed as reasonable, which implies that if it was conceived as of now, it would get an opportunity of making due in the middle with a neonatal unit experienced in thinking about untimely infants. An untimely infant conceived at 28 weeks (almost three months ahead of schedule) and thought about in an emergency unit an incredible possibility of endurance.

Most moms start to feel their children move at about this time. Feeling the baby inside you will be a little uncomfortable at first. Numerous ladies sense rippling developments (called enlivening) at around 16 to 20 weeks. Infant moving is only felt by a small number of women in this stage. Some believe its simply gas (and perhaps you ate an excess of bean stew) — yet in all likelihood, it's the infant. Around 20 to 22 weeks, fetal developments are a lot simpler to recognize, yet regardless they aren't predictable. Throughout the following month, they fall into an increasingly customary example.

**Dressing in maternity clothing**

Numerous ladies anticipate shopping for maternity garments, while others intend to remain in their typical garments for the entire length of time that conceivable. The maternity clothes are worn only for some months and working on these recommendations will help you make the right decision regarding maternity clothing:

✓ Don't prepare; purchase garments just as you need them. Envisioning how large you'll become and whether you'll convey the infant high up in your midsection or down low is troublesome. At the point when you do shop, purchase garments that fit serenely yet have enough space to suit further development.

✓ Don't be timid about tolerating pre-worn stuff. Women mostly tear away from their pregnancy clothes. Your companions are presumably glad to see their garments get more use.

✓ Look for relegation shops, recycled stores, and carport deals. They're great spots to discover modest maternity garments.

✓ If you experience difficulty discovering maternity garments in your style, recall that you can frequently go far through your pregnancy in ordinary stockings and enormous shirts or sweaters. (Joanne never needed to purchase any maternity garments whatsoever.)

✓ Perhaps the most significant things to purchase are agreeable shoes and roomier bras. Both shoe size and bra size can increment during pregnancy.

✓ You don't need to wear uncommon maternity clothing — except if you discover it particularly agreeable. Numerous sorts of normal underwear, particularly the swimsuit kind, fit well under a swelling tummy.

Various infants have distinctive development designs. You may see your child will in general move more around evening time — maybe to set you up for all the restless evenings you'll have after he is conceived! Or then again you may essentially be increasingly mindful of the child's developments around evening time since you're progressively inactive around then. When this is your second or third kid, you may begin to feel developments half a month sooner.

By 22 weeks, the baby will start to move and if you are not feeling this sensation, let the expert know. The ultrasound is the most common response to this situation, as this will help you know what is wrong with the child. When the placenta is embedded to the uterus, it creates a barrier between the child and the skin and the child's heartbeat cannot be gauged. The placenta goes about as a pad and defers when you first feel developments.

Following 26 to 28 weeks, if you quit feeling the infant move as much, of course, call your expert. By 28 weeks, you should feel development, in any event, multiple times an hour after you have supper. If you aren't sure whether the child is moving ordinarily, rests on your left side and check the developments.

## Understanding Your Changing Body

By 12 weeks, your uterus starts to emerge from your pelvis. At that point every week, your uterus develops by around one centimeter (1/2 inch). Numerous ladies start to appear at about four months, albeit looking pregnant shifts a lot. A few ladies look pregnant at 12 weeks; others aren't clear until 28 weeks.

A considerable lot of the progressions you experience have little to do with your midsection's size. Or maybe, they include your infant's improvement and your body's proceeding with adjustment to pregnancy. You may encounter a few, none, or every one of the side effects in this segment.

### Distraction and awkwardness

Until she was pregnant, you never would have accepted that losing keys, chancing upon furniture, and dropping things could be genuine reactions of pregnancy. We don't know about any restorative clarification for these impacts; however, a few ladies do feel they're increasingly harebrained and cumbersome. If you are forgetting things and making clumsy mistakes, do not worry about it. Now you have a reason for having overlooked your closest companion's birthday. This clumsiness will end when you will give birth to your child.

**Gas**

You may find that you build up the irritating and humiliating propensity to burp and pass gas at unfavorable occasions during this trimester. (Presently you can duel it out with your significant other.) If it's any relief, you're not the principal pregnant lady to run into this issue. Shockingly, however, you can do next to know about it — other than getting a pooch to accuse. Attempt to abstain from getting blocked up since that can exacerbate the situation. Likewise, abstain from eating enormous dinners that may leave you feeling enlarged and awkward or nourishments that you know exacerbate the issue even.

**Hair and nail development**

While you're pregnant, your fingernails and toenails may get more grounded than they've at any point been previously and develop at a phenomenal rate. Nail treatments are protected when done in a respectable, clean salon and frequently calm pressure, so kick back and make the most of your excellent nails!

Pregnancy likewise accelerates hair development. Sadly, a few ladies discover hair additionally starts developing in uncommon spots — all over or stomach, for instance. Waxing, culling, or shaving the undesirable hair is sheltered, however, hair evacuation creams (depilatories) contain synthetics that haven't been widely examined. Since more secure options are promptly accessible, we recommend evading these creams. Breathe easy in light of the probability that the undesirable hair will vanish after your infant is conceived.

**Acid reflux**

Indigestion — the consuming sensation you feel when stomach acids ascend into your throat — is normal during pregnancy. Indigestion has two fundamental causes (neither of which approves the old fantasy that acid reflux implies your child will have a ton of hair). To start with, the significant level of progesterone your body is delivering can slow assimilation and loosen up the sphincter muscle between the throat and the stomach, which typically counteracts the upward development of stomach acids. When the uterus is developing, this can push the stomach acids to the mouth.

You may get alleviation from acid reflux by following these recommendations:

✓ Eat little, visit dinners instead of huge ones.

✓ Carry a stomach settling agent when you're away from home.

✓ Carry a bundle of dry wafers to chomp on when you feel indigestion. They may kill the gas.

✓ Avoid hot, greasy, and oily nourishments.

✓ Avoid a lot of pop, caffeine, and espresso.

✓ Avoid eating just before sleep time, since acid reflux happens most promptly when you rest.

✓ If your acid reflux is getting painful, ask the doctor to prescribe a medicine. There are many medications that are safe to use during the pregnancy. The utilization of famotidine (Pepcid), ranitidine (Zantac), and omeprazole (Prilosec/Nexium) in the main trimester have been considered, and scientists found no expanded hazard for birth abandons, preterm work, or issues with fetal development. (The first trimester is the time of most serious hazard, so prescriptions demonstrated safe for use in the main trimester are probably sheltered in the subsequent trimester, as well.)

**Lower stomach/crotch torment**

Somewhere in the range of 18 and 24 weeks, you may feel a sharp agony or a dull hurt close to your crotch on either of the two sides. At the point when you move rapidly or stand, you may see it decline, and it might blur if you rest. This agony is called round tendon torment. The agony happens because as the uterus develops, the tendons stretch. The torment can be very awkward and, in some cases, can leave you speechless, however, it's ordinary. Fortunately, it as a rule leaves — or possibly decreases significantly — after 24 weeks.

At some point in the subsequent trimester (the specific time differs), you may begin to feel gentle, fleeting compressions or issues. These are alluded to as Braxton-Hicks constrictions and are nothing to stress over. They frequently are progressively perceptible when you're strolling or physically dynamic and afterward leave when you get off your feet. If they become awkward and standard (more than six out of 60 minutes), call your expert.

**Nasal clog**

The expanded blood stream that happens during pregnancy can likewise cause stuffiness and some growing of the mucous layers inside your nose. This can prompt postnasal dribble and, eventually, an interminable hack. Nasal saline drops may give some alleviation and are superbly sheltered to use during pregnancy. Keeping the air in your home or office very much humidified likewise makes a difference. Nasal showers and decongestants work, as well, yet abstain from utilizing these prescriptions for more than a couple of days one after another. You (or your partner, particularly) may see that all of a sudden, you're wheezing more than ever! This basic side effect again identifies with the expansion in nasal blockage. Our recommendation? Purchase your partner a decent arrangement of earplugs!

**Nosebleeds and bleeding gums**

Due to the higher volume of blood flowing through your body to support your pregnancy, you may encounter some bleeding from little veins in your nose and gums. This bleeding normally stops independent from anyone else, yet you can help by applying slight pressure to the point of bleeding. When you feel that the bleeding is getting serious, you need to contact your doctor. Utilizing a milder toothbrush may limit bleeding when you brush your teeth.

**Skin changes**

The hormones coursing through your body may cause abnormal things to happen to your skin. These changes, don't happen in all ladies, and if they do transpire, they have confidence they for the most part blur away after the child is conceived.

✓ You may see a dim line, called the linea nigra, on your lower midriff running from your pubic bone up to your navel. This line might be progressively perceptible in ladies with moderately dull skin. Reasonably cleaned ladies frequently don't build up this line by any means.

✓ The skin all over may likewise obscure in masklike dissemination around your cheeks, nose, and eyes. This obscuring is called chloasma or the veil of pregnancy. Sun presentation makes it significantly darker. Utilize a facial cream with sun square to limit the impacts of the sun on chloasma.

✓ Red spots, called arachnid angiomas, may abruptly show up anyplace on your body. Press on them, and they most likely turn white. These spots are convergences of veins which is formed by the increased estrogen. They'll most likely vanish after conveyance.

✓ Some ladies see a rosy shading on the palms of their hands. Known as palmar erythema, this shading is another estrogen impact, and it, as well, will leave.

✓ Skin labels (little, kind skin developments) are additionally a typical event and there is no clear evidence of why they are formed. Luckily, they, as well, blur away or vanish after pregnancy. Since they're probably going to determine in time, you don't have to hurry to the dermatologist to have them evacuated, except if they're extremely annoying.

**Checking In: Prenatal Visits**

In the subsequent trimester, you're probably going to see your professional about once like clockwork. At each visit, he checks your weight, your circulatory strain, your pee, and the fetal pulse. You might need to raise any inquiries you have about fetal development, labor classes, weight gain, and any unordinary side effects or distresses you may have.

Your expert routinely plays out various tests during your subsequent trimester to see if you're in danger for such difficulties as diabetes, paleness, or birth surrenders. You may likewise have an ultrasound test, with the goal that your expert can see things, for example, regardless of whether you're having twins, whether your infant is developing ordinarily, and whether you have a lot of amniotic liquid.

# Perceiving Causes for Concern in the second trimester

In this area, we talk about specific issues that can create during the subsequent trimester and indications that you ought to examine with your expert.

## Bleeding

A few ladies experience bleeding in the subsequent trimester. Potential causes incorporate a low-lying (placenta previa), untimely work, cervical inadequacy, or placental suddenness. Once in a while the specialist can't discover a reason. If you do encounter bleeding, it doesn't really mean you will have a premature delivery, yet you should call your primary care physician. Regularly he prescribes you have an ultrasound test and be checked to ensure that you're not contracting. Bleeding may expand the hazard for pre-experienced conveyance, so your primary care physician may prescribe that your pregnancy goes under extra-close reconnaissance.

**Fetal variation from the norm**

Although by far most of the pregnancies continue regularly, around 2 to 3 percent of babies are brought into the world with some variation from the norm. A large portion of these irregularities is minor, albeit some lead to huge issues for the infant. Some are because of chromosomal issues, and others originate from the irregular improvement of organs and structures. For instance, a few infants may have heart imperfections or anomalies of the kidneys, bladder, or gastrointestinal tract. A large number of these issues, however not every one of them, can be analyzed on a pre-birth ultrasound test. When stood up to with any such issue, the most significant initial step is to assemble all the accessible data about it, so you recognize what's in store and what the treatment alternatives are. Remember that even authorities may not be capable to let you know everything to expect until your child is conceived and they can additionally assess the circumstance.

**Inept cervix**

During the subsequent trimester, for the most part somewhere in the range of 16 and 24 weeks, a few ladies build up an issue known as an uncouth cervix or cervical inadequacy. The cervix opens up and widens, even though the lady feels no compressions. This condition may prompt the unnatural birth cycle. Surely, a bumbling cervix is regularly analyzed after the unsuccessful labor happens and, as a rule, couldn't have been anticipated. A lady who builds up this condition commonly doesn't see any side effects, albeit now and again she may report feeling pelvic greatness or weight that is strange, or she may see some spotting. Most ladies who experience an uncouth cervix do as such for no recognizable explanation. Some other danger issues are:

✓ Cervical injury: Some proof recommends that different D&Cs (enlargement and curettage) or techniques called cervical cone biopsy or LEEP (in which a cone-molded segment of the cervix is expelled in the finding or treatment of cervical variations from the norm) can expand the danger of cervical ineptitude. A critical tear of the cervix during an earlier conveyance may likewise build the hazard for cervical ineptitude.

✓ Multiple incubations: Some obstetricians accept that conveying different children, particularly triplets or more, may expand the hazard for an incompetent cervix. This issue is dubious; a few obstetricians prescribe setting a cerclage (a join in the uterus — see the clarification that follows) in all patients with triplets or more, yet others play out the method just in patients they believe are at high hazard for the inept cervix. A few patients who have experienced a strategy called multi-fetal pregnancy decrease may likewise be at an expanded hazard for clumsy cervix, albeit routine cerclage situation isn't suggested for them right now.

✓ Prior history of the inept cervix: After you have had a clumsy cervix, your danger of having it again in a consequent pregnancy is expanded.

The cerclage is generally put at 12 to 14 weeks, even though it's at times executed as a crisis strategy later in the pregnancy. Specialists most generally play out the method in the clinic under spinal or epidural anesthesia, however, the lady is typically released later that day.

A few ladies with a cerclage see they have an overwhelming release all through pregnancy. When you have a cerclage, let your physician know about how dynamic you can be. Entanglements related to crisis cerclage incorporate contamination, withdrawals, crack of films, bleeding, and unsuccessful labor. Similar entanglements can happen with elective cerclage, yet they're irregular.

**When you need to start looking for help!**

Coming up next is a rundown of second-trimester manifestations that require some attention.

- ✓ Bleeding
- ✓ An uncommon feeling of weight or greatness
- ✓ Regular constrictions or solid cramping
- ✓ Absence of typical fetal development
- ✓ High fever
- ✓ Severe stomach torment

## For Dads: Watching Mom Grow

Proceed with caution when making comments about your partner's paunch size. Possibly you are simply attentive, however, it's an incredible method to get the brush off without meaning it!

Appreciate the subsequent trimester. Regularly, it's the best time for some portion of pregnancy for the two guardians. Morning ailment blurs away, exhaustion dies down, and your partner starts to feel the infant move around inside her. Regularly, you, as well, can feel the child move by setting your hand on the mother's guts.

During this trimester, numerous moms get an ultrasound test to check the child's life systems. Attempt to come to see the ultrasound test (; it's one of the most agreeable pre-birth tests. You get the chance to see the child's hands, feet, and face, and you get the opportunity to watch the infant move around. Just because you see the living, moving, developing minimal human inside, and all of a sudden, the entire endeavor appears to be a great deal more genuine!

Before the second's over trimester, you may start pre-birth classes. Try not to rationalize! Go with your partner! The classes are intended for both dad and mother. During this time, you can discover how to be valuable during work and conveyance. What's more, you can likewise pose inquiries about what to envision — to alleviate your very own portion uneasiness.

## **A Short message from Mommy's Angels:**

Hey, are you enjoying the book? I'd love to hear your thoughts!

Many readers do not know how hard reviews are to come by, and how much they help an author.

I would be incredibly thankful if you could take just 60 seconds to write a brief review on Amazon, even if it's just a few sentences!

>> Click here to leave a quick review

Thank you for taking the time to share your thoughts!

Your review will genuinely make a difference for me and help gain exposure for our work.

# Chapter 7:
# The Last Three Months of Pregnancy

*You will learn*

---

*Preparing Yourself for The Delivery*

*Understand the Home Stretch*

*Knowing When You Should Be Concerned About the Delivery*

*Understand When to Go to The Hospital*

---

You're at long last prepared for the third trimester— your pregnancy's last trimester.

At this point, you're presumably familiar with having a jutting stomach, your morning affliction is a distant memory, and you've generally expected and appreciate the sentiment of your infant moving around and kicking inside you. In this trimester, your infant keeps on developing, and your expert keeps on observing you and your infant's wellbeing. You additionally start getting ready for the fresh introduction, which may mean anything from preparing to withdraw from nonappearance from your business to taking labor classes (or generally discovering what's in store during work and conveyance).

## Your Baby Gets Ready for Birth

At 28 weeks, your infant gauges around 14 inches (around 35 cm) and weighs around 21/2 pounds (around 1,135 grams). However, before the finish of the third trimester — at 40 weeks, your due date — it quantifies around 20 inches (50 cm) and gauges 6 to 8 pounds (around 2,700 to 3,600 grams) — now and then more, a few times somewhat less. The sensory system is developed during the third trimester. Apart from this, different the organs will start to take final shape during this time. The arms and legs get chubbier, and the skin gets thicker and smooth.

During the third trimester, your child is less defenseless to diseases and to the unfavorable impacts of meds; however, a portion of these specialists may, in any case, influence its development. The most recent two months are normally spent preparing for the progress to life on the planet outside the uterus. The progressions are less emotional than they were from the get-go; however, the development and development that happen now are significant.

By 28 to 34 weeks, the hatchling, for the most part, expects a head-down position (called a vertex introduction), like in Figure 7-1. Along these lines, the rump and legs (the bulkiest pieces of its body) possess the roomiest piece of the uterus — the top part. In around 4 percent of singleton pregnancies, the infant might be situated rear end down (breech) or lie over the uterus (transverse). (See the area "Perceiving Causes for Concern" later in this section for additional on the breach introduction.)

By 36 weeks, development eases back, and amniotic liquid volume is at its greatest level. After this point, the measure of amniotic liquid may begin to decay since bloodstream to the child's kidneys diminishes as the placenta ages, and the infant creates less pee (and accordingly less amniotic liquid). Truth be told, most professionals routinely check the amniotic liquid volume on ultrasound or by feeling your guts during the most recent couple of weeks to ensure that a typical sum remains.

**Movin' and shakin': Fetal developments**

Look down at your paunch during times of fetal action during the third trimester, and it might give the idea that an outsider from space is doing an aerobic move inside you. There is a change in the nature of the baby's development in the last phase. Close to the finish of pregnancy, fetal developments may feel less like pokes and increasingly like tumbles or rolls, and you see longer times of calm between developments. The hatchling is adjusting to a progressive infant-like the example, taking longer snoozes and having longer dynamic cycles.

A few ladies find that they go for times of feeling less fetal development, however then the developments get again and are ordinary. This is exceptionally normal and isn't a motivation to be concerned. In this last cycle, it is dangerous when you feel fetal developments in a short span of time. When it happens, you need to contact your gynecologist.

When there is a chance that your fetal developments may not commence at the right time, it is advised that you keep a journal that highlights fetal graph development. You can follow fetal developments in a few distinct manners. One route is to rests on your left side after supper to tally fetal developments and record to what extent it takes to check 10 developments. Another method for doing the test is to tally fetal developments while resting for an hour every day (it doesn't need to be that hour consistently) and to plot the number of developments on an outline given to you by your expert. This technique will help you to understand child development at different times.

BABY DROP

ISCHIAL SPINES

MOMMY'S ANGELS
EDITORIAL STAFF
GROW YOUR TODDLER TO THE BEST!

**Utilizing the breathing muscles**

Hatchlings experience are called the musical breathing developments from 10 weeks ahead, even though these developments are considerably more continuous in the third trimester. The baby doesn't really inhale, yet its chest, stomach divider, and stomach move in an example that is normal for relaxing. You don't see these developments, yet a specialist can watch them with ultrasound.

Numerous specialists accept these developments are signs that the infant is faring admirably. During the third trimester, the measure of time an embryo spends playing out the breathing development increments, particularly after dinners.

**Hiccupping in utero**

Now and again, you may feel a brisk, cadenced example of fetal developments, happen ring like clockwork. These developments are hiccups. A few ladies feel fetal hiccups a few times for the duration of the day; others sense them just seldom. Periodically, you may really observe the infant hiccupping during an ultrasound test. These hiccups are normal. They may feel weird, yet remaining on your head and drinking water, which we hear is an extraordinary fix, most likely isn't your best alternative at this point.

## Staying aware of Your Changing Body

As the child develops, so does your gut! Albeit huge is lovely, it can get awkward. You may see that your uterus pushes up on your ribs, and now and then you see kicking in one spot specifically — that is presumably where the infant's furthest points are either feet or arms. In case you're pregnant with twins or more, the distresses are, obviously, considerably progressively articulated. Ladies with twins may feel one infant move more than the other, which is normally identified with the children's positions — one infant might be situated with the arms and legs looking out and the other with them looking in. Regardless of whether you have one, two, or more infants inside, you see that moving around like you used to turn out to be increasingly more troublesome as you get greater.

## Accidents

When you are pregnant, you might have to face different issues related to balancing and working overtime. Don't stress if you experience a fall. Odds are great that the infant stays all around ensured inside your uterus and inside its sac of amniotic liquid, which is a brilliant regular pad. Be that as it may, just to be cautious, told your specialist. She may need you to come in to watch that the child is fine.

After a fall, the pain in the stomach can be very excruciating. When you feel bleeding of the amniotic liquid, this is the time when you need to contact your doctor. The doctor will conduct some tests to ensure that the baby is safe after the fall.

## Braxton-Hicks

You will feel that the uterus is changing in size during the later parts of pregnancy. When this happens, you might be having Braxton-Hicks constrictions. You need to contact the doctor when you are facing pain in the uterus. These contractions are probably are rehearsing contractions and are different from the one that you feel in labor.

**A pregnant lady knows no outsiders**

You may find that your midsection has all of a sudden become open property. Immaculate outsiders feel constrained to put their hands on your guts and disclose to you how satisfied they are that you're going to have a child! Albeit a few ladies locate this sort of conduct minding and supportive, others think that it is irritating, humiliating, and awkward. Cordially advising individuals not to contact your gut If they're making the move is alright.

Numerous individuals think of it as superbly obliging additionally to remark on your appearance. They may reveal to you that you look excessively fat or excessively slim; that you're conveying excessively wide or all in your posterior. "Hold up, you should be about prepared to pop!" they may scream, or "wow, you're pregnant!" For sure, the absolute best suggestion we can offer is that you don't give others a chance to make you insane. They may have the best of goals, yet they once in a while acknowledge how their words sound to you.

It is recommended to contact the doctor when you are having issues while pregnancy. So, don't stop for a second to ask your primary care physician or another social insurance supplier if what you hear stresses you. Yet, in addition, recollect what you know: If somebody discloses to you that you look excessively little, reveal to her your specialist estimates you with each visit to ensure that your alright development astute. When the ultrasound shows that the size of the baby is normal, you do not have to worry about anything. Your expert can generally promise you that your gut is measuring splendidly typical.

Numerous ladies feel constrained to reveal to all of you the awfulness accounts of their own pregnancies — or all the pregnancy frightfulness stories they've at any point heard. If you give an excessive amount of consideration, you'll just endure nervousness and unnecessary stress. Simply tell the individual respectfully that you truly favor not to hear her story (except if, obviously, you wouldn't fret these accounts).

**Carpal passage disorder**

The carpal passage disorder is the one in which you feel the blockage of blood in the body and your body shivers from time to time. It happens when expanding in the wrist puts pressure on the middle nerve, which goes through the carpal passage from the wrist to the hand. It can occur in one or two hands, and the agony might be more regrettable around evening time or after arousing. Carpal passage disorder is more typical in ladies who are pregnant than in the individuals who aren't a direct result of the expanding that accompanies pregnancy.

On the off chance that carpal passage disorder gets tireless or troublesome, talk about it with your professional. Wrist supports, accessible at some medication stores or careful stockpile stores, can soothe the issue. Make an effort not to be debilitated if it doesn't appear to show signs of improvement during pregnancy, however, because it normally improves (regularly significantly quick) after conveyance.

**Weakness**

The weakness you felt right off the bat in your pregnancy may return in the third trimester. The weakness occurs because you have additional weight in your body and the constant anxiety can also take toll on your body and mind. The women who have having second or third pregnancy may feel more tiring because they have more children to take care of.

You need to stay relaxed when you are pregnant. Do as little work that you can do and do not worry about the work that is left behind. Set aside effort for your-self and get as a lot of rest as you can. Agent errands. At whatever point conceivable, let others help with family unit errands and different duties. Do what-ever you can to exploit the peaceful occasions. You need to know that your responsibilities will increase after the delivery, so this is probably the best time to give your body some rest.

**Hemorrhoids**

Nobody needs to discuss them, however, hemorrhoids — enlarged, swollen veins around the rectum — are a typical issue for pregnant ladies. They're basically varicose veins of the rectum (we talk about varicose veins later in this segment). The augmenting uterus causes hemorrhoids by pushing on significant veins, which prompts the pooling of blood, and at last causes the veins to amplify and expand. Progesterone loosens up the veins, enabling the growing to increment. Obstruction exacerbates hemorrhoids. Stressing and pushing hard during defecations puts included to weight the veins, making them extend and potentially jut from the rectum.

This bleeding doesn't hurt the pregnancy, yet if it gets a visit, converse with your primary care physician and perhaps observe a colorectal master or general specialist. Sometimes the treatment of hemorrhoids becomes important and this your doctor will tell you about the best course of action in this matter. In the interim, you can attempt the accompanying:

✓ Avoid obstruction Straining to push out hard stool can exacerbate hemorrhoids.

✓ Exercise. Action expands entrail motility, so the stool doesn't get excessively hard.

✓ Stay on your feet and stay active. Doing so mitigates additional weight on your veins.

✓ Try over-the-counter topical prescriptions, for example, Preparation H or Anusol, or steroid cream. Numerous ladies discover some help with these drugs.

✓ Take steaming showers a few times each day. Absorbing warm water can help diminish the muscle fits that regularly cause the torment.

✓ Use over-the-counter hemorrhoidal cushions, (for example, Tucks) or witch hazel cushions to clean and cure the territory. These cushions frequently give a cooling, relieving help.

Pushing during the second phase of work can aggravate hemorrhoids or cause them to show up where they weren't previously.

**Insomnia**

Having a comfortable sleep when you are pregnant becomes difficult as times. Finding an agreeable position when you're eight months along isn't simple.

You feel similar to a stranded whale. Getting up five times each night to go to the washroom doesn't make things any simpler. Be that as it may, you may discover alleviation in the accompanying:

✓    Drink warm milk with nectar. Warming the milk discharges tryptophan, a normally happening amino acid that makes you tired; the nectar makes you produce insulin, which likewise makes you lazy.

✓    Exercise every day. Movement tires you out, which implies you'll nod off sooner.

✓    Go to bed somewhat later than expected. You'll invest less energy attempting to nod off.

✓    Limit your fluid intake after 6 p.m. Try not to constrain it to the point that you become got dried out, in any case.

✓    Invest in a body cushion. You can take care of it around your body different spots, making it simpler to locate an agreeable position. You can get a body pad in practically any retail chain.

✓    Take a warm, loosening up shower. Numerous ladies state a shower helps make them feel sluggish.

**Feeling the infant "drop"**

During the prior month conveyance, a lady may see that her stomach feels lower and that all of a sudden, it's simpler to relax. This drop is felt when the baby drops to the pelvis. This development is likewise called helping. It commonly happens a little while before conveyance in ladies who are having their first youngster. The women who are pregnant for the second or third term may not feel the baby drop.

When dropping occurs, you may find that you're all of a sudden considerably more agreeable. Your uterus doesn't press up on your stomach or stomach as much as it used to, so breathing is simpler, and indigestion may improve. Simultaneously, in any case, you may feel more weight in your vaginal zone — numerous ladies feel largeness there. A few ladies report feeling abnormal, sharp twinges as the infant's head moves and apply pressure on the bladder and pelvic floor. Having the infant "drop" doesn't anticipate when work will occur.

You may not see that you have dropped. During your pre-birth visit, the child's head can be located with the help of many tests. The fetal head is considered at the right position when it is at the same level of the ischial spines. A simple test can help you to know if it is at the right position or not.

At the point when the fetal head is at the same height as the ischial spines, it's at zero station. Most specialists isolate the pelvis into diving stations from − 5 to +5 (albeit some utilization − 3 to +3).

Regularly toward the start of work, the head might be at − 4 or − 5 stations (genuinely high — here and there called gliding, because the fetal head is as yet coasting in the amniotic pit). Work continues until the head drops right to +5 when the conveyance is going to start.

It is known that when the head is at this position, chances of the normal delivery increases. Doctors will surely recommend vaginal delivery when the baby's head is locked in the place. The locking of the head is a good sign, but this does not ensure the vaginal delivery process. Your doctor will not know till the delivery time whether the baby will be delivered via the vaginal route or they need to make a cesarean delivery. In case you're having your subsequent youngster or more, the infant's head may not connect with until well in the process of childbirth.

**Pregnancy rashes and tingles**

Pregnant ladies are dependent upon similar rashes that nonpregnant ladies get. One rash is interesting to pregnancy, be that as it may. It is called Pruritic Urticarial Papules of Pregnancy, or PUPP. It sounds terrifying, however, it's extremely even more a disturbance than everything else because it can cause some serious tingling. It happens all the more regularly during a first pregnancy and in quite a while having twins or more (the more hatchlings, the more noteworthy the probability).

PUPP will, in general, happen late in pregnancy and is portrayed by hives or red fixes that initially show up in the stretch blemishes on your guts. These patches can spread to different zones on the mid-region and to the legs, arms, chest, and back. They never spread to the face. (Thank paradise for little supports.) fortunately, the condition represents no hazard to the infant. Infection can be formed when you are pregnant and the doctor will suggest a simple blood test to make sure you are free of all infections and other types of diseases.

The main surefire approach to make PUPP leave is to convey. A few ladies disclose to us that the tingling leaves inside long periods of conceiving an offspring. Skin creams containing Benadryl can likewise help, however, these items can at times dry the skin, which just exacerbates the tingling. A few ladies get help from taking Benadryl orally, however, check with your primary care physician before doing as such. At last, in exceptionally extreme cases (which are uncommon), the specialist may endorse a transient course of steroids or different prescriptions.

Regardless of whether you don't have a rash, you may see that you tingle a great deal, particularly where stretch imprints create. You may feel tingling when you are pregnant and it is completely normal because the child is growing in your belly and causes the skin to stretch. When you are pregnant, there is a small chance that the bile acids in the blood will increase. This increase in the bile acids will cause tingling in the body. Reports show that only two percent of women have this problem during their pregnancy. Skin creams and oral medications can be used to treat this problem. On the off chance that the tingling is serious, your PCP may prescribe oral meds that help to clear the bile acids from the circulation system. A few examinations have proposed that the child ought to be checked with non-stress tests (see Chapter 8) when the mother has this condition since it is related to an expanded danger of confusion. The tingling leaves not long after conveyance, however, the condition may repeat in future pregnancies.

**How to Plan for breastfeeding**

You need to know that the mother's milk is very healthy for the child. When you are planning to start breastfeeding, you need to make sure that you talk to the doctor about your medical condition and also find ways to tighten your areolas. Otherwise, they will become sore when you are breastfeeding your child. Since split areolas can be excruciating, setting them up diminishes any inconvenience you may have. You can attempt delicately scouring or kneading your areolas between your fingers, presenting them to air, scouring them tenderly with a wash material, or wearing a nursing bra with the folds down so your areolas rub against your garments. Creams and oils neutralize, toughening, so don't utilize them on your areolas.

A few ladies stress that they don't have the correct sort of bosoms for bosom encouraging, however, no bosom type is correct or wrong. Bosoms both enormous and little can create sufficient milk. A few ladies with withdrawn or upset areolas can make breastfeeding simpler by kneading their areolas so they project more. Some maternity or child stores sell uncommon bosom shells that utilization suction to enable the areolas to turn out.

Numerous ladies see from at an opportune time in pregnancy that their bosoms event partner emit a yellowish release. This release is colostrum, and it's what the infant sucks out and swallows in the initial not many long stretches of life before genuine milk comes in. Colostrum has a higher protein and lower fat substance than milk; above all, it contains antibodies from your invulnerable framework that help ensure your child against specific contaminations until her own resistant framework develops and can dominate.

A woman should not worry when they do not create colostrum when they are planning to breastfeed; not creating colostrum not the slightest bit implies that you won't deliver satisfactory milk. Every lady is extraordinary; some hole from the bosoms during pregnancy and some don't. Regardless of whether it isn't self-evident, your infant will, in any case, get colostrum the initial not many occasions she breastfeeds.

**Sciatica**

A few ladies experience discomfort stretching out from their lower back to their posterior and down one leg or the other. This pain is not a regular, deadness is known as sciatica since it's because of weight on the sciatic nerve, a significant nerve that branches from your back, through your pelvis, to your hips, and down your legs. You can soothe gentle instances of sciatica with bed rest (move from side to side to locate the most agreeable position), steam showers, or warming cushions applied to the agonizing zones. Consulting with the doctor is always a great idea when you are worried about your medical condition.

**Brevity of breath**

You may find that as pregnancy continues, you become progressively shy of breath. The hormone progesterone influences your focal breathing focus furthermore, may cause these sentiments of windedness. Besides, as your extending uterus presses upward on your stomach, your lungs have less room to grow regularly. (When Joanne was pregnant with her subsequent kid, she used to be so shy of breath that the main books she could peruse to her little girl were ones with short sentences. Dr. Seuss needed to sit on the rack until after she delivered it.)

Much of the time, the brevity of breath is impeccably ordinary. Chest problems may arise when you deliver the baby for the first time. A woman is not ready to breastfeed the child and consulting with the doctor and finding a suitable solution is the best option you have.

**Tackling Stretch imprints**

It is nearly impossible to avoid the stretch imprints when you are pregnant. You can stay away from the stretch imprints by some ways. You can do some research on the internet to find the ways to deal with stretch imprints. Your skin stretches to suit the broadening uterus and weight gain, causing the stretch imprints. A few ladies most likely additionally have some hereditary inclination for stretch imprints. The imprints commonly show up as pinkish-red streaks along the stomach area and bosoms, yet they blur to shimmering dark or white a while after conveyance. Their accurate shading relies upon your skin tone — they seem browner on dull cleaned ladies, for instance.

No cream or salve is totally viable in forestalling stretch imprints. Numerous individuals believe that scouring vitamin E oil on the gut averts stretch checks or encourages them to blur quicker, however, the adequacy of vitamin E has never been demonstrated logically. Avoiding unnecessary weight gain is one of the best ways to keep your body in great shape when you are pregnant. The weight gain can also affect the health of the child.

**Planning for Labor**

Close to the finish of your third trimester, you're probably going to ponder conveyance and foresee what that will resemble. Huge numbers of our patients need to know when their work may begin and whether they can do anything to impact the planning or to expedite it sooner. Going into labor is one of the most stressful times for the first-time moms and in this section, we will highlight some of the most important things that you need to know when you are pregnant and also provide information about the cesarean delivery process. We highlight all the major topics in a way that you can feel ease about the entire process and deliver your first baby with ease.

## VAGINAL DELIVERY

**a.** Dilation of the cervix and breaking of amniotic sac

**b.** Delivery of the head

**c.** Delivery of the body

**d.** Delivery of the placenta

**MOMMY'S ANGELS**
EDITORIAL STAFF
GROW YOUR TODDLER TO THE BEST!

## Making labor preparation

When you are in the last trimester, the doctor will announce the birth plan and this plan will help you understand the labor and delivery process. Your emotions will be very high when you are about to deliver the baby. A rush of emotions will fill your days and staying calm will help you to avoid any rash decisions when you are pregnant. This birth plan will help you in many ways and you will get to know how your will deliver the baby, how you can bear the pregnancy and labor pain and also highlight all the underlying procedures of vaginal and cesarean delivery. You might have many assumptions leading up to the day you are about to deliver and this birth plan ensures that you at ease with this process.

For instance, a few clinics have managed about fetal heart observing during work. The most significant piece of a birth plan — be it composed or verbal — is to give a stage that encourages an open dialog among you and your supplier about your inclinations in any place there is a decision.

It all boils down to the day you are about to give birth to the child. We urge you to be in constant communication with the doctor and the clinic where you are planning to give birth.

**Requesting a C-Section**

Many like to make a C-section delivery and they request their doctors to do so. According to the statistics, more than 2.5 percent deliveries in America are made via C-section upon the request of the patient. It is advised that you understand the dangers and advantages of the C-section delivery. A doctor will most likely help you understand the process and ensure that you are make a knowledgeable decision when it comes to vaginal and cesarean delivery. If you are planning to have more children in the future, having a cesarean delivery is not a good option because of its dangers. Women who are afraid of the vaginal delivery pain mostly opt for the cesarean delivery. Having a vaginal delivery is a normal and safe process and the doctors only recommend the cesarean delivery when there are some complications during pregnancy.

The potential advantages of this method of conveyance are a lower danger of baby blues drain and a lower danger of urinary incontinence. The last has been demonstrated to be valid in the primary year after conveyance, however, after that time, the danger of this issue is equivalent between mothers who convey vaginally and the individuals who have cesarean conveyance on request.

The drawbacks to cesarean on request are a more extended remain in the clinic, transient breathing issues for the child, and greater dangers in your resulting pregnancies for issues like uterine burst.

## Perceiving Causes for Concern

During the last many long periods of pregnancy, you see your expert more frequently than previously. In any case, certain inquiries and issues may emerge between visits. Everything begins to warm up during the later phases of the third trimester, with both the infant and your body planning for conveyance. Here is a portion of the key things that may lead you to call your PCP.

**Bleeding**

If you experience any huge bleeding, let your professional know right away. Some third-trimester bleeding is innocuous to you and your infant, however once in a while, it can have genuine ramifications. Persuading assessed to be certain all is well bodes well. Potential reasons for third-trimester bleeding incorporate

✓   Preterm work: This is characterized as having constrictions and changes in the cervix before you're 37 weeks along.

✓   Inflammation or disturbance of the cervix or the innocuous bleeding of a shallow vein on the cervix: Either of these can happen after intercourse or after a pelvic test.

✓   Bloody appear: This show is generally not exactly the measure of blood you would see during a typical menstrual period, and it's regularly blended in with mucous. See Chapter 10.

**Breech introduction**

A child is in a supposed breach position when its hindquarters or legs are down, nearest to the cervix. A lady's danger of having a breach child diminishes the further along she goes into her pregnancy. (The rate is 24 percent at 18 to 22 weeks yet just 8 percent at 28 to 30 weeks. By 34 weeks, it's down to 7 percent, and by 38 to 40 weeks, 3 percent.) If your primary care physician decides your infant is in a breech position during your third trimester, she will talk about your alternatives, including vaginal breech conveyance (which is once in a while done nowadays), outside cephalic adaptation, or cesarean segment.

## EFFACED DELIVERY

CERVIX · STEP 1 · STEP 2

STEP 3 · STEP 4, 100% EFFACED

**MOMMY'S ANGELS**
EDITORIAL STAFF
GROW YOUR TODDLER TO THE BEST!

**Diminished amniotic liquid volume**

The therapeutic term for diminished amniotic liquid volume is oligohydramnios. (It likewise used to be called dry birth.) It might be found on a normal ultrasound, or your PCP may presume it just by feeling your uterus. This condition can happen in relationship with intrauterine development confinement (see the later segment "Fetal development issues"), preterm crack of the films, or different conditions, or the reason may not be recognizable. Typically, a mellow reduction in an amniotic liquid is anything but a significant reason for concern; in any case, your expert starts to screen you all the more intently — with non-stress tests and ultrasound tests — to ensure that no issue emerges. In case you're near your due date, your specialist might need to convey the infant. Then again, in case you're just 30 weeks along, the best alternative might be expanded rest and close perception. Obviously, the administration of the issue additionally relies upon its motivation.

**Fetal development issues**

You may discover at a routine pre-birth visit that your specialist thinks your uterus is estimating either too enormous or excessively little. This finding isn't a reason for the prompt alert. Frequently in this circumstance, your specialist proposes that you have an ultrasound test to show signs of improvement thought of how large the infant is. Ultrasound is utilized to gauge portions of the infant — the head's size, the stomach area's periphery, and the thighbone's length. Your expert at that point connects these estimations to a numerical condition that gauges the fetal weight (EFW).

The child's weight is also an important factor that determines the safety at the time of the birth. It is rare that the child's weight will pose a problem in the pregnancy and there are certain ways by which the doctors can ensure a safe delivery despite of the abnormal weight. So, this is something you should not be worried about and always trust your physician to make the right decision.

Remember that although ultrasound is a magnificent apparatus for evaluating fetal development, it isn't great. Deciding the child's weight by an ultrasound test isn't equivalent to putting the infant on a scale. Weight evaluations can shift by as much as 10 to 20 percent in the third trimester because of varieties in body pieces. So, if your infant is outside the ordinary range, do not stress.

If your child gauges enormous (macrosomia), your expert may propose you have another glucose screen to check for gestational diabetes. Sometimes the fetal development is slow and the child's weight and growth is slowed. Additional ultrasound tests before the delivery will help the doter to pursue the course of action that will ensure a safe delivery.

**Releasing amniotic liquid**

If you see your clothing is wet, a few clarifications are conceivable. It might be a little pee, vaginal release, the arrival of the mucous module the cervix, or real spillage of amniotic liquid (otherwise called break of the layers). Frequently, you can determine what it is by looking at the liquid. The mucous release will, in general, be thick and globby, while the vaginal release is whitish and smooth. Pee has a trademark smell and doesn't stream consistently without your exertion. Amniotic liquid, then again, is regularly clear and watery and frequently is lost in spurts. Some of the time you have a major spout of water when films burst, however if the layer has just a little gap, the spillage might be meager.

If you spill what you think might be amniotic liquid, summon your specialist right or go into your emergency clinic for assessment. If the liquid is grisly or greenish-dark colored, make certain to tell your specialist.

The greenish liquid may mean the infant has had defecation (meconium) inside the uterus. More often than not, such an occasion doesn't demonstrate an issue, yet once in a while, it implies the child is being pushed. Your specialist ensures the child is alright by checking the infant's pulse (generally by playing out a non-stress test).

## Preeclampsia

Preeclampsia, in which hypertension is related to the spilling of protein into the pee and once in a while growing (edema) in the hands, face, and legs, is a condition one of a kind to pregnancy. Preeclampsia (likewise called toxemia or pregnancy-prompted hypertension) isn't extraordinary; it happens in 6 to 8 percent all things considered. It can go from being extremely gentle to being a genuine ailment.

Preeclampsia, for the most part, goes ahead progressively. Your professional may from the outset see just a slight rise in your circulatory strain. Preeclampsia can happen suddenly and a doctor will help you to deal with this problem in an effective manner. You will have to make frequent visits to the doctor. When you are facing this issue, the doctor will advise you to lie on your side more often.

## Understanding Preterm work

Preterm work is when a woman has compressions in her cervix before she reaches her 37 weeks mark. Numerous ladies have constrictions however no cervical change — in which case it isn't genuine preterm work. What's more, your expert decides how regularly you're shrinking by putting you on a uterine compression screen

The withdrawals related to preterm work are ordinary, diligent, and regularly awkward. They normally begin feeling like awful menstrual issues. (Braxton-Hicks withdrawals, interestingly, aren't standard or steady, and they normally aren't awkward.) Preterm work may likewise be related to the expanded mucous release, bleeding, or spillage of amniotic liquid. Diagnosing preterm work as right on time as conceivable is significant. Drugs planned for capturing untimely work best if the cervix is enlarged under 3 centimeters. If work happens following 35 weeks, your professional most likely won't attempt to stop your compressions aside from in uncommon conditions.

# Chapter 8:
# What to expect from Labor process

*You will learn*

---

*Finding out what is labor process*

*Understanding the Stages of Labor*

*Manage Childbirth Plan*

*Determining the right birthing method*

---

We are still baffled about the labor and delivery process. No medical advancements have been able to solve this mystery. Labor may be activated by a blend of upgrades produced by the mother, the infant, and the placenta. Many experts believe that different biochemical and steroid are the cause of the delivery. Since we don't know precisely how labor begins, we additionally can't pinpoint precisely when it will happen.

This section encourages you to perceive the indications of labor and discloses to you what's in store at every one of the three phases of labor. It likewise addresses such significant issues as labor acceptance, torment the board, the checking of your infant's wellbeing, and elective birthing strategies.

## How to know if Labor is real or not!

It is normal to feel fake labor pain when you are in the last trimester. This is your body's way to prepare yourself for the delivery. You can never be certain of when you are about of give birth. Even the women who are giving birth for the second time may not be able to know if they are going to give birth today. This area causes you better recognize your own labor (yet despite everything you may wind up considering your professional a few times or in any event, making numerous outings to the clinic or birthing focus, just to discover that what you believe is work truly isn't).

You may encounter a portion of the early side effects of labor before this actually starts. As opposed to demonstrating that you're in the process of giving birth, the accompanying indications recommend that work may happen decently soon. There is no certain time for when you will experience this labor pain of feelings related to labor. Some women only feel this sensation for a few hours before birth while others feel it for days before giving birth. In rare cases, some women feel labor like sensation even week before they are about to conceive. When you are in the dynamic labor phase, it is best to be in constant contact with the doctor. You should not rush to the hospital when you feel the labor pain.

**Seeing changes before labor starts**

As you close to the finish of your pregnancy, you may perceive certain progressions as your body plans for the enormous occasion. You may see every one of these side effects, or you may not see any of them. Once in a while the progressions start a long time before work begins, and here and there they start just days prior:

✓       Bloody appear: No, the wicked show isn't the most up to date blood and gore movie by Wes Craven. As changes in your cervix occur, you may remove a few mucous releases blended in with blood from your vagina. The blood originates from little, broken vessels in your cervix.

✓       Diarrhea: A pregnant women will discharge prostaglandins for some days before of labor. This may cause diarrhea in pregnant women.

✓       Dropping and commitment: The baby may drop in the pelvis a couple of weeks before you are about to conceive. This will create some difficulty in pregnant women. Some tightness may be felt in the vagina and its nearby areas. The pain is mandatory but you can ask your doctor to find some ways to control the pain. The uterus may also lower which will relax your body. This process helps a pregnant woman to give birth easily.

✓       Increase in Braxton-Hicks withdrawals: You may see an expansion in the recurrence and quality of Braxton-Hicks compressions. There are many women who will feel these withdrawal days before they are about to give birth.

✓       Mucous release: You may emit a thick mucus release known as the mucous fitting. This mucus will help to hold your cervix in position and the uterus will be saved from different infections. As your cervix begins to disperse (destroy) and widen in anticipation of conveyance, the attachment may cleanout. Try not to stress; losing your attachment doesn't mean you're inclined to contamination.

## What is real and fake labor

Recognizing genuine labor from bogus labor isn't in every case simple. In any case, a couple of general qualities can assist you with deciding if the indications you're encountering mean you're in the process of giving birth.

The fake labor affects most of the women. Women who are giving birth for the first time are not sure about the labor process and these tips will help them identify the fake labor from the real labor. It is the fake labor is the constrictions disappear suddenly or have unpredictable repetitions. Now, you must be wondering how would you know if you are having a real labor. When the withdrawals last for more 60 seconds and they are more frequent in nature, this is the time when you are having a real labor.

At the point when you land at the emergency clinic, your primary care physician, a medical caretaker, a maternity specialist, or an inhabitant doctor plays out a pelvic test to decide if you're in the process of giving birth. The specialist likewise may connect you to a screen to perceive how frequently you're contracting and to perceive how the fetal heart reacts. In some cases, you discover immediately whether you're really in the process of giving birth. In any case, the professional may need to hold you under perception for a few hours to see whether the circumstance is evolving.

You're viewed as in labor in case you're having standard compressions and your cervix is changing decently quickly — destroying, enlarging, or both.

## Understanding when you need to see the doctor

It is recommended to keep track of your labor contractions. You need to contact your doctor when you feel that you are about to give birth. It is completely fine to have a false call related to labor and there is nothing to be ashamed about. You need to make sure that you note the time of your withdrawals for some hours and check their repetitions. These repetitions will increase when you are about to give birth. When the withdrawals are frequent and they happen every 5 to 10 minutes, this is the perfect time to call the doctor. When you are having passed the 37-week mark and are feeling compressions, do not wait and call the doctor right away. This is not the time to note the compression time.

Call your professional when:

✓ Your constrictions are coming nearer together, and they're getting progressively awkward.

✓ Having your water break may come as a limited quantity of watery liquid spilling out, or it might be a major spout. If the liquid is green, dark-colored, or red, let your expert know immediately. Passing meconium doesn't really demonstrate anything isn't right, however, it can infrequently be related to fetal pressure.

✓ You're not feeling a sufficient measure of fetal development

✓ You have steady, serious stomach torment with no help between constrictions.

**Checking for work with an inner test**

The doctor will do some internal tests when you are about to give birth. The tests are conducted to find the following things:

✓    Dilation: After dynamic work starts, the pace of cervical enlargement accelerates, and the cervix expands to 10 centimeters before the finish of the primary phase of work. Frequently, you're viewed as

✓    Position: When work starts, the child regularly begins looking to one side or right side. As work advances, he pivots until the head accepts a facedown position with the goal that the child turns out taking a gander at the floor. Every so often, the infant pivots to the contrary position and turns out just right, taking a gander at the roof.

## The main characteristics of Labor

Any individual who conveys babies realizes very well that work can generally amaze you. As specialists, we may anticipate that a lady should convey rapidly and find that her work takes quite a while, while another lady, whom we think will take perpetually, may convey quickly. In any case, in most by far of pregnant ladies, work advances in an anticipated example. It goes through effectively recognizable stages at a genuinely standard rate.

Your professional can keep tabs on your development through work by performing interior tests at regular intervals. How effectively you progress through work is estimated by how rapidly your cervix widens and how easily the hatchling drops descending through the pelvis and birth waterway.

Specialists become worried over the advancement of work if it's excessively moderate or if the cervix quits widening and the hatchling doesn't slip. They have a short-hand framework for portraying the factors that decide how effectively a lady clears her path through work: the three Ps (traveler, pelvis, and power). As it were, the infant's measure and position (the traveler), the pelvis' size, and the constrictions' quality (the power) are extremely significant variables.

For conveyances after the first, work is usu-partner shorter (around 8 hours). Work is partitioned into three phases, depicted in the accompanying areas.

**The main stage**

The main phase of work happens from the beginning of genuine work to full enlargement of the cervix. It is partitioned into three stages: the early (inert) stage, the dynamic stage, and the change stage. Each stage has its own one of a kind attributes.

**The early or dormant stage**

You will feel the compressions every 20 minutes in the dormant phase of labor. The compression time will be reduced to every five minutes when you are about to give birth. You will feel the compressions for about 60 seconds and as you are close to give birth, these compressions will last for more than 90 seconds. The cervix size will also increase when you are in the labor. You will feel the expansion of about 3 to 5 centimeters. When you are giving birth for the first time, this dormant stage will last for more than 7 hours and the stage time will reduce as you are giving birth for the recurring times.

You may feel pain when in this stage. Some women do not feel any pain in this stage and this feels more like the menstrual issues. This is the time when you need to be in the hospital as you can give birth anytime now. The doctor will make sure that you are in a comfortable position and will keep you under observation during this time.

At an opportune time in this stage, you might be generally agreeable at home. You can take a stab at resting or dozing, or you might need to remain dynamic. A few ladies discover they want to clean or play out some other family tasks. In case you're eager, eat a light feast (soup, squeeze, or toast, for instance), however not an overwhelming one — if you later need anesthesia to manage work entanglements. You might need to time your constrictions, yet you don't have to fixate on it.

If you begin to turn out to be increasingly awkward, the withdrawals happen with more recurrence or force, or your films crack (your water breaks), call your specialist or go to your clinic.

Numerous ladies discover strolling around makes them progressively agreeable and diverts them from the agony during the early piece of work. Others want to rest in bed. Ask your specialist whether your medical clinic has any limitations on strolling during work.

**Dynamic stage**

This phase lasts much shorter than the initial phase and it is more predictable than its former stage. When you are giving birth for the first time, this stage will last for more than five hours. The compressions will be recurring and may last for 60 seconds. You may feel compressions every 3 minutes in this stage. In this stage, your cervix will enlarge by 9 centimeters.

A pregnant woman may feel a lot of pain in this stage. Spinal pain is the main problem that you will face in the dynamic stage. The position of the child may cause pain in the back of the body. When the baby is facing the back instead of the front, then you may feel the pain known as back labor pain.

Most women are admitted to the hospital at this stage. Depending on your condition, you may either be stuck on the bed. The patients who are not feeling pain may stroll for a while to ease their minds. You need to make sure that you follow the instructions of your doctor at this stage. If the doctor asks you to stay in bed, you should not plan to walk. At this time, the breathing exercises that you have learned during the labor classes will come handy. You need to be in constant communication with the doctor at this stage. You need to discuss what your body is going through or if you are feeling any pain during this stage. Staying relaxed is the key to easily pass this stage. You need to know that you might feel some pain during this stage but it is essential that you don't get anxious about the delivery process.

**First stage**

The time frame of the first stage is something that is not easy to calculate. You will feel withdrawals every 2 minutes and these withdrawals will last for more than 60 seconds. The compressions or withdrawals at this stage are very serious. The cervix of the pregnant woman will expand to about 10 centimeters. If you have the desire to push the baby, you need to discuss it first with the doctor. The doctor will guide you in the best way to push and how you can experience less pain in the delivery process. For some women, breathing exercises can help a lot. You need to indulge in the breathing exercises when you are about to give birth. The pain medications can also help during this time, but they need to be used after consultation with the doctor.

**Potential issues during labor's first stage**

Most ladies experience work's first stage with no issues. In any case, if an issue emerges, the accompanying data sets you up with the data you have to deal with it with a reasonable, centered personality:

✓ Prolonged inactive stage: Your professional will be unable to decide when labor really begins, so knowing without a doubt when work becomes drawn out isn't in every case simple either.

At the point when an expert discovers that work is taking excessively long, he reacts in one of two different ways. One methodology is to utilize medicine, for example, a narcotic, to enable you to unwind. Work may then die down (which implies that it was bogus work from the start), or dynamic work may start. The two methodologies are canvassed in more detail before in this section.

✓ Protraction issue: Protraction issue can happen if the cervix enlarges too gradually or if the child's head doesn't plunge at a typical rate.

You will know that the second stage of labor has started when your cervix is expanded up to 10 centimeters. You may be in the second stage for more than an hour when you are delivering the baby foe the first time. This time will consequently reduce when you are giving birth for the second time. This stage is also known as the pushing stage. After this, you will enter the third stage of delivery. In this stage, the delivery of the placenta happens. The stage usually lasts for 15-20 minutes.

# Chapter 9:
# Bringing The Baby In the World

*You will learn*

---

*Understanding Vaginal Delivery*

*Preparing for the cesarean delivery*

---

At the point when you're approaching the end of the second phase of labor, you're near the point of delivery. Remember that you don't need to stress a lot early. You can set yourself up — by taking labor classes and by perusing this book, for instance. Furthermore, recollect that your specialist and his or her aides in the delivery room will control you through the procedure. Acknowledge and depend on their assistance. Trust in yourself, as well, and let this common procedure move along with extra special care.

Fundamentally, babies are delivered in one of three different ways. The first way by which a baby is delivered is through the vagina with the help of waterways that push the baby out. The second way of delivery is also through the vagina but with the help of vacuum extractor. The third way is a little bit complicated and is known as cesarean delivery. The doctor will help you choose the process by which a baby is delivered. The delivery process depends upon the medical history of the patients and also the pelvic size of the woman. You should not feel anxious if the doctor suggests the cesarean delivery. In this section, we will discuss all these parts and how you should prepare yourself for a healthy delivery.

## Understanding the Vaginal Delivery

Women usually think that they will have a child in the 40$^{th}$ week of pregnancy and it will be delivered via vaginal route. This is not possible for all pregnant women. In case you're having a child just because, it might appear to be really startling. Regardless of whether you've had a kid previously, stressing a piece until you see your lovely child is ordinary. A little information goes far, however, and being educated and arranged for all potential outcomes is constantly useful. Most likely, you'll experience what specialists call an unconstrained vaginal delivery, which implies that it happens because of your pushing endeavors and continues without a lot of intercessions. When the baby is not passing through the vaginal route, the doctors will make use forceps to hold the baby's head or may use vacuum extractor to deliver the baby. When one of these things are used to deliver the baby, this type of delivery is known as employable vaginal delivery. We spread the two courses of occasions in this section.

During the primary phase of labor, your cervix widens and your films rupture. You will reach the principal phase of labor when your cervix is expanded by almost 10 centimeters. You will feel a lot of weight on your pelvis and rectum when you are about to give birth via vagina. You might also feel like defecation when you are in this phase. The defecation sensation will also be felt during the final withdrawals or compressions. This sensation is caused when the baby is passing through the vaginal route with the help of waterways.

When the doctor uses epidural during the vaginal delivery, you will not feel this sensation. Epidural is the local anesthesia that is used to remove the pain from the delivery process. The pain is usually caused when you have reached the expansion limit of the cervix. At this time, the doctor will ask you to push the baby out. Your medical attendant or specialist per-structures an inside test to affirm that your cervix is completely enlarged. If it is, she instructs you to begin pushing.

Regardless of whether your medical attendant, specialist or birthing specialist is really training you during pushing shifts from emergency clinic to the emergency clinic and from professional to expert. A pregnant woman needs to be at a certain resting position so that the baby can be delivered easily. The doctor will analyze your position and ensure that the baby's head is dropped at the right moment.

**Pushing the baby**

The time of pushing the baby differentiate. It takes an average of 30 minutes to an hour to push the baby out. In rare cases, it may take up to 3 hours in this process. The time depends upon the size of the baby's head and its position within the body. Having epidural may help you to ease this pain. The process takes a lot of time when you are delivering the baby for the first time. When you are giving birth for the second time, the pelvic muscles may expand long before your due date and it will only require a little effort to deliver the baby. Your medical attendant or professional gives your explicit directions on the best way to push. While you're pushing, your infant moves more remote along its descending course. Ladies regularly start pushing when the infant's head has plummeted into the pelvis. The time and effort required to push the baby out depends on the position of the baby. After you convey the head, your PCP may guide you to quit pushing, so she can suction some liquid out of the child's mouth, and furthermore feel to check whether the umbilical line is around the infant's neck. From that point onward, you'll push a couple of more occasions to deliver the remainder of the child.

You have a few potential situations wherein to push.

✓ Lithotomy position: This is one of the most common positions to push the baby out. In this position, you have to lie on the bed and lift up your knees to your chest. Simultaneously, you twist your neck and attempt to contact your jawline to your chest. You need to form a C with your body. This position might not be comfortable for you but this helps to ease your butt and uterus and make the delivery process an easier one.

✓ Squatting position: In this position, the earth's gravity will help you to push out the child. This position may ease the delivery process but you cannot hold this position for a long time.

✓ Knee-chest position: This position is recommended for those women who have issues delivering the baby via squatting and lithotomy position. The knee-chest position might be ungainly for certain ladies and hard to remain in for exceptionally long.

**Getting an episiotomy**

When you are about to give birth to the child, the baby's head will stretch your skin. The doctor will make a small cut in the skin to assist the delivery process. Some doctors suggest that the episiotomy is unnecessary when delivering a baby. It is a good thing that you understand the vaginal delivery process as this helps you to stay calm during this important event of your life. You should expect having an episiotomy when you are delivering the baby for the first time. This is a normal procedure and can make the deliver process easier. You should discuss having an episiotomy with your doctor when you are in the labor.

The kind of episiotomy made may rely upon your body, on the situation of the infant's head, or on your expert's judgment. Specialists can browse two primary kinds of episiotomies:

√ Median: In this type, the small cut is made from the vagina to the butt.

√ Mediolateral: In this type of episiotomy, the small cut is made in the opposite direction of the butt

If you are not being given epidural, a small sedative can be given to you to numb the nearby area. A middle episiotomy might be less awkward later on, and it might mend all the more effectively.

Your expert analyzes the birth waterway cautiously after delivery and closes up any slashes that should be fixed. These slashes, for the most part, mend rapidly and never cause long haul issues. Try not to stress over having the lines evacuated — most specialists utilize the sort of sutures that disintegrate without anyone else.

## Taking care of delayed second-arrange labor

You need to understand that if you are in the second phase of labor for more than two hours, it is termed as delayed labor. There might be complications that you have to face when you are in the delayed labor phase. However, all these complications can be easily tackled by a proficient doctor. When the baby's head is not the right position or it is not aligned with the lady's vagina, this is when you might have to face the issues of delayed labor. Now and then, the child's head is in a place that squares further drop. The doctor will ensure that the child's head is in the right position or they will make you change your position so that the delivery process can go as smoothly as possible. You may likewise take a stab at changing your situation to push all the more successfully. Now and again, forceps work (see "Helping Nature: Operative Vaginal Delivery," for more information on this topic. As a last resort, your primary care physician may prescribe a cesarean delivery.

## The defining moment: Delivering your infant

At the point when the child's head stays unmistakable between constrictions, your medical doctor will get you into a position to convey. The hospital staff will place the leg bolsters in front of you so that you can easily give birth to your child. No matter if you are giving birth in a delivery room or in the birthing room, the doctor will make sure that you are in a comfortable position to push the baby out. Delivering the infant is a very complicated process and the doctor will walk you through this process when you are about to give birth.

When you are pushing out the baby, the medical staff will regularly clean the vaginal area so that the kid can be conceived easily. This also acts as the lubricant. Mostly iodine solution is used to clean the area. The decision to do the episiotomy is made in the last few minutes of the delivery. When you push out the baby, the baby head is in the loose position and the doctor will ask you to stop pushing when the baby's head is out of your body. If the baby's head is stuck in the vaginal channel, the doctor will use a vacuum extractor to pull out the baby.

**Delivering the placenta**

The third part of the delivery focuses on the delivery of the placenta. The placenta is also known as the fetal membrane. This stage endures just around 5 to 15 minutes. Despite everything you have compressions, however they're a lot less extraordinary. With the help of these compressions, the uterus will be separated from the placenta. After this detachment happens and the placenta arrives at the vagina's opening, your expert may request that you give one progressively delicate push. Numerous ladies, elated by and depleted from the delivery, give little consideration to this piece of the procedure, and later on, don't recollect it.

**Fixing your perineum**

The perineum is the place between the rectum and the vagina and when you have successfully delivered the placenta, the doctor will examine your vagina and perineum. The perineum may be damaged during the pregnancy and the doctor will analyze the place and provide the suitable fix. A sedative may be used to numb the place so that you do not feel any pain when the doctor is fixing this place. When all the fixing procedure is completed, the medical staff will clean the part. The medical staff will remove the legs from the rest and provide you cover. After you have delivered the baby, you might feel some compressions, and these compressions help in stopping the bleeding.

**Helping Nature: Operative Vaginal Delivery**

When the baby's head is not in the perfect position for delivery and the doctor thinks that some additional help is required, they use forceps or a vacuum extractor to proceed with the delivery. This is a perfectly normal way to deliver the baby. The forceps and vacuum extractors are sterilized ensuring that you do not get any infection. This process is known as operative vaginal delivery. This is safer than cesarean delivery and the forceps nor the vacuum extractors will harm your baby.

Such a delivery might be fitting to utilize when

✓ You've pushed for quite a while, and you're too worn out to even think about continuing pushing sufficiently hard to deliver.

✓ You've pushed for quite a while, and your expert figures you won't convey vaginally except if you have this kind of help.

✓ The infant's pulse design shows a need to deliver the child very fast.

✓ Sometimes the baby's position is not perfect for delivery and this prompts the doctor to use these instruments.

With the vacuum extractor placed on the top of the baby's head, the doctor gently pulls out the baby. The vagina can only be stretched to a certain position and with the help of these instruments; you will not have to push the baby hard. When the doctors plan the vaginal delivery and the baby is almost at the end, these instruments make it easy to conceive. You need to know that it is up to the doctor to select one of these instruments to perform delivery. Truth be told, these methods can regularly assist ladies with maintaining a strategic staying away from cesarean delivery (however not generally — see the following area). A doctor needs to be experienced in handling these instruments carefully. You need to stay relaxed during the delivery and do breathing exercises to ensure a safe delivery. Many doctors will make additional room with the help of episiotomy when they have to use these instruments to make a delivery. The doctors will also give you additional tranquilizers to help with the pain when they ought to use this method to deliver the baby. When the doctor has applied these instruments for delivery, they will ask you to push the baby out. The vacuum extractors and the forceps are generally used when the baby's head is stuck in the vagina and the rest of the delivery is mostly completed by pushing. You might have some imprints when these devices are used to perform the delivery. The vacuum extractor is applied on the round part on top of the baby's head and this procedure does no harm to the baby. This imprint, as well, leaves in a couple of days.

## Understanding Cesarean Delivery

You should not worry if you need a vaginal or cesarean delivery. The cesarean delivery is only recommended if the child is not in the right position or if you have medical problems. The cesarean delivery may cause some complications for the first-time mothers and if you are medically fit, you should not request a cesarean delivery. The choice of the delivery procedure rests on the doctor and you should understand the complications and benefits of all types of delivery procedures before the labor. The decision of the delivery procedure is made in the final hours of the delivery so do not worry about it beforehand. You also need to know that cesarean is a surgical procedure and this procedure may take longer than the normal vaginal delivery. After a medical caretaker or attendant's associate cleans the patient's guts with the disinfectant arrangement, a medical attendant spots clean sheets over the patient's stomach. One of the sheets is raised to make a screen with the goal that the eager guardians don't need to watch the technique. (Even though labor is typically an encounter shared by the two guardians, a cesarean delivery is as yet a careful activity. Most specialists feel that the methodology isn't something that eager guardians should watch since it includes surgical tools, bleeding, and introduction of interior body tissue that is ordinarily not seen, which is upsetting to numerous individuals.)

Numerous medical clinics enable the mentor or partner to remain in the working room during cesarean delivery, however, this choice relies upon the idea of the delivery and on emergency clinic arrangement. When the doctor is doing the cesarean delivery, there might be some compilations. In case of any dangers, the doctors rush to save the mother and baby. Your attendant cannot be in the surgical room.

**Getting anesthesia**

Epidural and spinal are one of the most used anesthesia during the cesarean process. Both this anesthesia will numb the bottom part of your body and help you stay conscious during the procedure. You may experience some kind of pulling during the procedure but will feel no pain. The process may take some time and the doctor will walk you through all the processes before they start operating you. In some rare cases, the doctors may use general anesthesia. All things considered, there is a high success rate in case of cesarean delivery so you should not be worried about anything.

All things considered, you're snoozing during the cesarean and absolutely ignorant of the system. Likewise, general anesthesia might be required sometimes in light of entanglements in pregnancy that make it incautious to put epidurals or spinal.

**Taking a gander at purposes behind cesarean delivery**

The reasons your PCP may play out a cesarean delivery are many (see the rundown later in this area). Yet, all are tied in with delivering the baby in the most secure, most beneficial way that could be available while likewise keeping up the mother's prosperity. There are different reasons for choosing cesarean delivery. The delivery is either done when a woman has some medical problems and the baby cannot be delivered thought the normal vaginal route. The cesarean delivery ensures that the woman and the baby are healthy.

The doctor will guide you through the process of cesarean delivery and why it is important for you. If you choose the cesarean delivery by yourself, you have to ask everything about the process and if this will have any post effects on your body or not. When the baby is not present in the right position for vaginal delivery, the doctor will choose the cesarean delivery route. Discuss all the issues that you might have when you are having a cesarean delivery with the doctor when you are being transferred to the delivery room. There are complications in both vaginal and cesarean delivery. Both convey a few dangers, and regularly your professional asks you which dangers are generally adequate to you.

Do not panic if the doctor chooses to have a cesarean delivery at the last moment. Specialists and medical attendants are prepared to deal with these sorts of crises. The doctor will propose the cesarean delivery for many reasons. Following are the explanations behind elective, or arranged, cesarean delivery:

- Your baby is not in the correct position for vaginal delivery.
- You have medical issues such as placenta previa
- You will have to deliver the baby via cesarean procedure when you have pat medical procedures such as evacuation of uterine fibroids
- A cesarean delivery is necessary if you are expecting triplets or more

Purposes behind impromptu however nonemergency cesarean delivery:

✓ The doctor will have to move to cesarean delivery when the baby is enormous as compared to the pelvis of the woman and cannot pass through the vagina.

✓ Signs demonstrate that the child isn't enduring labor.

✓ Maternal ailments block safe vaginal delivery, for example, a serious heart ailment.

✓ Normal labor grinds to a halt.

Explanations behind crisis cesarean delivery:

✓ Bleeding is much.

✓ Prolonged easing back of the child's pulse.

There is no difference when the baby is delivered via vagina or it is removed from the woman's body by an incision in the uterus. You need to understand that the babies who are born via cesarean delivery do not have a cone-head. The baby will have a cone-head if you are having a delayed delivery. The main purpose behind the selection of the cesarean delivery is the safety of the mother and the child. The doctors will not recommend the cesarean delivery if the child can be born naturally. This surgery is common and a professional gynecologist can easily deliver a baby with the help of this procedure. According to the reports, almost 30 percent women require cesarean delivery for a number of reasons. The experts will analyze your medical condition and will only choose this procedure if this can result in a safe delivery of the child. Almost all surgeries have some dangers and the cesarean delivery is no exemption. Luckily, these issues aren't normal. The fundamental dangers of cesarean delivery are the development of disease in the bladder and uterus. There is also an increased danger of the excessive bleeding and some woman may also require blood transfusion. After the cesarean delivery, the woman may also face the issues of blood clusters in the pelvis and legs.

**Recovering from the C-section surgery**

Like other surgeries, it will take some time for you to recover. Medical staff will keep you under observation for some hours until you are in a stable condition. The time that you have to stay in the hospital depends on your medical condition and how well you are recovering. It is safe for you to hold and see your child during this time. You will be fully conscious but it will be difficult for you to continue your normal life.

You need to understand that the time needed to recover from the cesarean delivery is usually longer than the vaginal delivery. You will be asked to stay in the hospital for two to four days after your surgery. We will discuss different complications that you might face in the next chapter.

**Congrats! You Did It!**

Ladies may encounter different feeling after their children are conceived. The range of sentiments is really endless. More often than not, you're completely defeat with bliss when your hotly anticipated infant at long last is conceived. You might be unbelievably mitigated to see that your child seems solid and obviously alright.

Sometimes the child needs to go through different tests after they are born and you might not be able to see or hold them for some time. These tests will usually take some hours so do not get panic at this stage. The doctor will keep you posted about the condition of your child. Holding the child for the first time is a very alluring feel and this is why, women want to see their child as soon they are born. You need to keep a grip on your sentiments and wait for the doctor to conduct their tests. Simply take each minute in turn. You've gotten through a marvelous occasion.

## Shaking after delivery

Very quickly after delivery, most ladies begin to shake wildly. Your partner may imagine that you're cold and offer you a cover. Covers do support a few ladies, yet you aren't shuddering because you're cold. The reason for this marvel is misty, however, it's about widespread — even among ladies who have cesarean deliveries. A few ladies feel apprehensive about holding their children since they're shaking to such an extent.

Try not to be worried about this shaking. It, for the most part, leaves inside a couple of hours after delivery.

## Know more about postpartum bleeding

You might have to face some bleeding after you give birth to your child. This happens when the uterus contracts and get into its original place. Due to the contraction of the uterus, some veins in your body will crush and you may bleed.

If the uterus doesn't contract regularly, exorbitant bleeding may happen. When you have twins or triplets, the uterus may not contract in a timely fashion and may cause excessive bleeding otherwise known as uterine atony. There are many reasons that can cause uterine atony. You may have to experience uterine atony when some tissues of the placenta remain in the body after the placenta is delivered. Disease in the uterus may also cause this complication in first-time moms.

Of course, sometimes, unreasonable bleeding occurs for no obvious reason. Medical officer will do some therapeutic movements on your body to ensure that the bleeding stops. If the sessions do not help, the doctor will prescribe some medications that will help you stop bleeding. It is seen that the bleeding will stop after the delivery without any medicines. You should discuss the postpartum bleeding with your doctor and how you can help them minimize it.

**Hearing your child's first cry**

Not long after delivery, your child takes its first breath and starts to cry. This crying is the thing that grows your child's lungs and helps clear further discharges. Rather than generalization, most specialists don't hit an infant after it's conceived, however rather utilize some other technique to invigorate crying and breathing — scouring the child's back vivaciously, for instance, or tapping the base of the feet. Try not to be astounded if your infant doesn't cry the exact moment after it's conceived. Regularly, a few seconds, if not minutes, go before the child begins making that stunning sound!

**Checking your infant's condition**

The apar scores are used to check the condition of the child. These scores were developed by Dr. Virginia Apgar in 1952. These scores will help the doctors to check the condition of the child. The scores are determined after checking the baby's muscle tone, breathing, pulse, shading and muscle reflexes. If the baby's Apgar score is more than 6, they are considered healthy. Since a portion of the attributes is in-part subject to the newborn child's gestational age, untimely infants often get lower scores. Factors, for example, maternal sedation likewise can influence a child's score.

Numerous unseasoned parents tensely anticipate the aftereffects of their kid's Apgar score.

The motivation behind the Apgar score is simply to support your PCP or pediatrician distinguish babies who may require some additional consideration in the early infant time frame. Cutting the umbilical cord is the final stage of delivery.

In the wake of cutting the string, your professional either lay your child on your stomach area or gives the infant to your labor medical attendant to put under a newborn child hotter.

The decision relies upon your child's condition, your PCP's or medical caretaker's standard practice, and on the institutional strategy where you're delivering.

## Checking In: Baby's First Doctor Visit

Previously or after delivery, somebody from the medical clinic requests your pediatrician name. This specialist ought to be somebody who is approved to work at the medical clinic where you have delivered however might be a similar pediatrician you intend to use after you leave the emergency clinic. If you live, some good ways from the emergency clinic and have chosen a pediatrician near your home who doesn't have benefits at the medical clinic where you deliver, you still need another pediatrician to think about your infant during the medical clinic remain. Contingent upon the time you deliver, the pediatrician may see the child around the same time, or he may see the infant the following day.

The pediatrician arranges an assortment of standard blood tests and infant screening tests. The particular screens that are required differ from state to state yet frequently incorporate tests for thyroid malady, PKU (a condition in a tough situation utilizing some amino acids), and other inherited metabolic issues. The aftereffects of these screening tests normally don't return until after you take your child home. The pediatrician gives you the outcomes at your child's first office visit. If any of the tests return positive, the state additionally informs you via mail. Make certain to ask the pediatrician upon release when your child ought to be seen once more.

**Considering pulse and circulatory changes**

Recollect how your professional checked the fetal pulse during pre-birth visits? You may have seen then how quick the beat was. In utero, the infant's pulse is, 120 to 160 pulsates every moment, and this pulse pat-tern keeps during the infant time frame. Your infant's pulse additionally can increment with physical action and delayed down when he does.

After your infant is conceived, significant changes available for use happen. Ordinarily, this shunt closes on the primary day of life. Now and again, a mumble is heard in the principal days after the child is conceived, which demonstrates changes in bloodstream. This mumble, which is known as a PDA for patent ductus arteriosus, is typically ordinary and nothing to stress over. Be that as it may, some heart mumbles may require further examination — explicitly, an extraordinary sonogram, or echocardiogram, of the child's heart. In any event, when a cardiologist discovers mumbles because of little auxiliary issues (like a little gap in the heart's septum), numerous mumbles leave all alone. If your infant is determined to have a mumble, talk about it completely with the infant's pediatrician or a pediatric cardiologist who has some expertise in these conditions.

**Seeing weight changes**

Most babies get thinner during their initial hardly any long periods of life — ordinarily around 10 percent of their body weight — which, obviously, if you weigh just 7 or 8 pounds (3,200 or 3,600 grams), adds up to not exactly a pound (454 grams). This marvel is typical and is generally brought about by liquid misfortune from pee, dung, and sweat. During the initial hardly any long periods of life, the run of the mill newborn child takes in almost no nourishment or water to supplant this weight reduction.

Preterm babies lose more weight than full-term children, and it might take them longer to recover their weight. Conversely, pampers which are little for their gestational age may put on weight all the more quickly. For the most part, most new-borns recover their birth weight by the tenth day of life. By the age of five months, they're probably going to twofold their birth weight. Before the finish of the primary year, then triple it.

# Chapter 10:
# Dealing with Special Concerns

*You will learn*

---

*Problems in delivery*

*Solutions for pregnant mothers*

---

Women who are becoming mothers for the first time will be experiencing an entirely new thing in their lives. In the state of pregnancy, the woman has to be very careful to avoid any unfortunate event. The way of her living will be entirely different during the months of labor. She has to pay special attention to herself and her coming baby. Different factors can create complications for the pregnant women. You need to be aware that the medical conditions, age of the parents and the BMI have an impeding effect on the pregnancy and the health of the child. These things can create issues when during the labor phase as well.

## How Age matters in pregnancy

Giving birth to a baby is a tough job. The mother has to be medically stable and fine to undergo this process. When men and women are planning to become parents, they should consider their age and other relevant things. Women in their late thirties can face some problems in their pregnancy. Teen mothers also face different kinds of challenges during their pregnancies. Always seek medical advice before planning a baby.

**Becoming pregnant in age 30 or over**

Now the time has completely changed as most of the women prefer to get married and have children in their thirties. Those days are gone when ladies become pregnant in the early '20s or their teen ages. Presently, a large number of women post-pone having families until they've completed their education, and after that, they prefer to get settled in their professional career before getting married. That is why divorce is very common, and most of the women end up having kids with their second spouse — frequently when they're in the age bracket of the 30s or 40s (and some of the time 50s).

How old is excessively old? The appropriate response is when you arrive at menopause — or even a few years earlier. When your body never again delivers solid eggs that can be used to become embryos. There have been many advancements in the medical field and the processes such as Vitro fertilization can be applied to easily impregnate a woman. Even the older women can get pregnant with the help of this process. In this method, eggs are given by another woman are utilized.

There are many women who are concerned about the special issues that are faced by a pregnant woman. They need to know that at what age they need to worry about the special problems that are faced by women. The women fall into the advanced maternal age also known as AMA, when they are 35 years or older. (A casual term, however maybe less offending than the options that are likewise utilized: older gravida, matured gravida, and the especially sad old gravida.) Women who are older than 35 may have some chromosomal issues when they are pregnant. Pregnancy issues increase after the age of 35. Older women may have to face more pregnancy anomalies than younger women do.

Pregnancy issues may be higher in the older women but the babies born to these mothers are as healthy as the babies born to the younger women are. The mothers have the increased chance of developing pregnancy issues such as preeclampsia. The older woman also cannot withstand the dangers of cesarean delivery.

In any case, these dangers aren't high, and, much of the time, any issues that outcome are minor. Normally, an older lady's involvement in pregnancy depends entirely on her fundamental health. A lady of 48 years of age or even 50, having perfect health, can perform extremely well in the time of her pregnancy.

**Problems for old dads**

The issues related to genes also affect the older dads. These genetic difficulties make it difficult for older men to become fathers. Somewhat, pregnancies including more aged fathers, ought to similarly be singled out for perception. There is no outright age cutoff for "cutting edge fatherly age," however numerous individuals utilize 45 or 50 (some contend it ought to be 35, similarly all things considered for women).

As far as the issues in the older women are concerned, the primary cause of concern for the women older than 35 is the chromosomal abnormality. Men also face similar problems when they are older than 35; some problems with the gene mutation are related to dwarfism. Even a single mutated sperm can cause this issue in the child. This issue is also termed as a recessive genetic disorder. The doctors will conduct some tests that will help them determine the quality of the sperm.

**Too young to be a mother**

Teenage pregnancy in women raises a different kind of concerns. This age group doesn't continue any expansion in chromosomal abnormalities, and these ladies may encounter a higher rate of some congenital disabilities. Since young mothers are not exactly on ideal dietary routine, they additionally experience a higher occurrence of low-birth-weight babies. Young mothers are likewise at a greater danger of creating preeclampsia, have high chances of cesarean delivery, and are less chance of breast-feed. Because of their exceptional circumstances, young mothers need extra guidance and direction. In case you're a young mother, we urge you to get sufficient pre-birth care, to pursue a solid eating routine, and to consider the advantages of breast-feeding.

# Having Multiple Babies

It is simple and good to have twins or more babies at a time, to somebody who's never faced this truth. It's either "double pleasure at the same time" or a living bad dream (double the work and sacrificing half of your sleep). When you are having twins or triplets, you need to be ready to face some complications as well. The women who have been pregnant with twins can tell you all about the issues that you might have to face during your pregnancy. In case you are expecting triplets or more, the same principles that apply to twins mostly apply to triplets.

A woman's body is capable of giving birth to healthy babies at the same time, but a woman might have to face issues when they are giving birth to twins or triplets. The doctors will conduct different tests to ensure that women who are giving birth to the twins are healthy. Additional ultrasound tests are also required to ensure that the babies are growing at a normal pace. When you are having multiple babies, the family medical history also plays a vital role in determining the success of the labor. There are many women who produce more than one egg in the ovulation cycle. Your doctor must know the history of your family background especially if any twin birth happened at any time.

Twins can be either fraternal or identical. These good old terms don't totally portray how twins happen. Identical twins look particularly similar and are consistent with similar sex. Multiple babies come from the mating of a single sperm and a single egg. The egg is then divided into two parts which help in giving birth to twins. In rare cases, an egg can be divided into three parts giving birth to triplets. As the babies are conceived from a single sperm, they have similar likeness and habits.

On the other hands, fraternal twins are conceived when two sperms meet with two different eggs. As discussed earlier, some women produce two eggs in a single cycle and these two twins does not have the same characteristics and have different habits in general. You can see them as two different children of the same parents. They are conceived at the same time and can be of opposite sex. These dizygotic twins who emerge from two zygotes don't share an identical arrangement of genes.

After the age of 35, the chances of women having identical twins increase. The chance to conceive fraternal twins will decrease after this certain age. When the women have two ovulations at the same time, this means that they have a higher chance of giving birth to the fraternal twins. When women have a higher chance of twinning from the maternal side, there is a strong chance that she will give birth to fraternal twins. The genes and medical history of both parents also play a vital role in increasing the chance of conceiving the twins. It is not sure that the women will give birth to twins or not and it is determined in the first trimester.

## Differentiating multiples as identical or fraternal

Many women are confused about whether they are going to give birth to identical or fraternal twins. Identifying this is very easy, and you can ask the doctor or the ultrasound technician about this. The ultrasound technician or your primary care physician can tell: If the infants are of opposite genders, they're fraternal. The babies can be either fraternal or identical if they are from the same sex. Different ultrasound tests can help you identify the sex of the babies and also tell you if they are identical or fraternal.

When you are expecting twins, there are different scenarios that can affect the growth and type of twins that you are going to give birth to. If the egg splits in the first few days of fertilization, then you will have two fetuses and two different amniotic sacs. The term that is used to define such a phenomenon is called diamniotic. The ultrasound will confirm that the kids are fraternal and they will be formed from different eggs. When the eggs split in the third day or beyond, the babies will be formed in different amniotic sacs but they will have a single placenta. For this phenomenon, the egg has to split before the eighth day of fertilization. There are many reports that the kids who originate from different eggs may have the same characteristics. You will give birth to the monoamniotic kids when the egg splits between the 8 and 13 days of fertilization. This means that the kids will be in the single amniotic sac. Kids who are monoamniotic are most likely to be identical.

**Examining mothers with Down syndrome who have twins or more**

Women who suffer from down syndrome can also make perfect mothers. There was no clear test on determining the state of women with the syndrome. The only way for screening woman was to take their blood samples when they are almost four months pregnant. Identify the issues with common tests is not easy when you have twins or triplets in your belly. It will be difficult to find out if the fetus has down syndrome or not. Latest technologies such as nuchal translucency helps provide additional information on this topic and will highlight if the babies have down syndrome or not. With triplets or more, utilizing the nuchal-translucency estimation alone will, in general, be the most accommodating methodology since it's hard to decide how to utilize the mother's blood markers in this circumstance.

**Genetic testing**

You might have to face many complications finding out the issues such as amniocentesis and chronic villus when you are expecting multiple babies. One of the main issues that you will face is testing both embryos separately. As both embryos are connected in the early stages of pregnancy, the issue may worry some doctors. When you are expecting identical twins, both babies may have the same problem. If you identify a genetic variation from the norm (or absence of any genetic irregularities) in one, the equivalent is quite often valid for the other. Testing all the babies is important when you are expecting fraternal babies.

**Amniocentesis**

In the multi-fetal pregnancies, testing the mother for amniocentesis is very important. A simple test needs to be conducted and the doctor will insert a needle in all the fetuses to ensure the well-being of the baby. Under the direction of ultrasound, the amniocentesis is done. After the specialist expels some liquid from the principal fetus, she may leave the needle set up to infuse mischief less natural blue color (called indigo carmine) into that baby's amniotic sac. (Try not to stress, you won't be giving birth to a Smurf. This blue color is absorbed after some time.)

Chorionic villus examining, or CVS, is a bit complicated in multi-fetal pregnancies, but expert physicians are capable of handling the activity. You will notice that the CVS is not possible in some cases as the placenta is located in the same places. The mother will have the chance to get amniocentesis somewhat later in pregnancy (at around 15 to 18 weeks, as opposed to 10 to 12 weeks for CVS).

**Tracking the baby**

Your primary care provider assigns your infants. These empower your primary care physician to communicate with you and others (attendants and other restorative faculty) what every child is and to pursue the advancement of each infant independently and reliably all through pregnancy. This infant is generally brought into the world first. (A few patients assign their own smart names. We had one patient with twins who nicknamed her children Gucci and Prada before birth so she could monitor them.)

**How to tackle multiple pregnancies**

In case you are pregnant with multiple babies, do not overlook everything else we have written in this book. From different points of view, your pregnancy continues like some other. There are many issues that may accompany multiple pregnancies. You may face issues such as increasing belly and may be exposed to nausea and fever. The time taken to conceive the baby will also be increased. When you are pregnant with more than one baby, it will be difficult for the doctors to diagnose your body for pregnancy issues. You need to understand that there you will have to face more complications when you are pregnant with more babies. Below, we highlight a significant number of ways in which your experience might be fairly different:

- **Activity**: In the past times, specialists prescribed women with twins to bed rest for 24 to 28 weeks. Your body will go through more changes when you are pregnant with more than one baby. The activity of the woman ensures that the baby is healthy. The mother's activity needs to be reduced week by week and this ensures that the baby is growing perfectly. If you have developed premature birth or have issues with fetal development, your primary care provider may suggest you relax. With triplets or more, the advantage is not clear, but numerous obstetricians routinely prescribe bed rest beginning in the second trimester.
- **Diet**: when you are expecting more than a single baby, you need to increase your daily calorie intake. On an average a woman who is expecting twins should consume 300 extra calories than the mother who is expecting a single child. For triplets, the sky is the limit for them, no agreement exists, but clearly, your nutritional intake should be more than your previous routine to fulfill the needs of the babies.
- Folic acid: If you are pregnant with more than a single child, you need to understand that you can get iron deficiency. The daily requirement of the babies is different than a single child inside your body and this may also create an iron deficiency in your body. You may also have to face folic deficiency in the body. Folic and iron are the main components of hair and nails and due to this, many women start to lose hair when they are pregnant. doctors will prescribe some special supplements that will help them regain the lost iron in the body.

- Nausea: You need to know that you will be facing heavy bouts of nausea and vomiting when you are pregnant with more than a single child. The sickness will be severe in the first trimester and as will subside in the coming months. You will have increased pregnancy hormones in your body and they will cause this sickness. Fortunately, nausea and vomiting of moms carrying multiple babies are high as compared to moms of single infants.
- **Visits to doctors**: Your expert is probably going to pursue basically a similar routine she utilizes for moms of single children. On every visit to the doctor, the doctor will test your pee, pulse, heart condition and the condition of the babies. As you are pregnant with more than a single child, the doctor will call you for more visits. When you are pregnant with twins, the doctor will also test your pelvis to make sure that it is not expanding more than it should be. The internal organs will be tested via ultrasound as usual. If you are not experiencing any pain or awkwardness in the body, the doctor will not bother you with additional tests.
- **Ultrasound assessments:** Checking the fetal developments when you are having twins is very important. The doctors recommend multiple ultrasounds every month to ensure that the fetal growth is stable. These tests will also help to identify the issues in the fetal development as well. Timely identification of the issues will help the doctors to cure the disease in the timely fashion. When you expect a single child, the doctor can use the fundal height measurement to find the issues but with multiple embryos, this scenario cannot be

entertained. Women with multiple fetuses and expecting triplets may have underlying issues that need proper care. There is a chance of premature birth and the doctor will do transvaginal ultrasounds to explore the risk of premature birth.

- Weight gain: When you are expecting twins, there will a 15 to 20 kg weight gain. In any case, the precise weight you gain relies upon your pre-pregnancy weight. During the second and third trimester, you can expect to put up one pound of weight each week.

## Precautions at the time of labor and delivery

Understanding the labor process will surely help you stay calm during your pregnancy. The cesarean delivery is necessary when you are pregnant with three babies. The latest medical research highlights that if the babies and woman is healthy, then the delivery of triplets is also possible via vaginal route. Pregnancy goes easily for moms of twins, however, work and delivery can at present be mind-boggling. Special care is needed for women who are delivering triplets so it is necessary that the kids are delivered in the medical center where they can get proper care. Some additional work may be required so it is best that the medical staff is ready to take care of any complication that may arise. As there are multiple babies in your body, they might be in different position and hard to conceive. Essentially, their positions can be categorized as one of three conceivable outcomes:

- The position of the embryos is difficult to predict and the babies can take any position inside your body. There is a strong chance that the both the embryos are upside down. There is a good chance that the vaginal delivery is possible when the babies are in this position.
- Babies can take different positions in the body and there is no guarantee that the babies will be in the same position. In a scenario, one embryo may be facing the top while the other may be in the downward direction. In this case, you need to have a thorough discussion with the doctor about the delivery of the babies. The doctors will try their best of ensure that the vaginal route. Having an experienced doctor in this scenario will most likely be beneficial.
- There is a 20 percent chance that the babies will be in the transverse position. As the previous condition, the doctor will have to deal with these mixed positions and based on their experience, they will choose the best route for delivery.

**Issues which can be faced by mothers with multiples**

You need to be in close observation when you are pregnant with two or more babies. The multi-fetal pregnancies are always difficult to handle and the doctors need to take extra care when dealing with such cases. The following points are considered to be important when taking care of the mother. Try not to give this rundown a chance to scare you. It is best to identify the issues in the early stages as this will help the doctor to prepare for the procedure in a proficient manner.

**Preterm conveyance**

Premature delivery is one of the main causes of concern with mothers who are pregnant with more than one child. As we have discussed earlier, it takes approx. 40 weeks for a child to born. When you are pregnant will twins, you will give birth in around 36 weeks. The time gets even less when you are pregnant with triplets. It takes approx. 33 weeks for triplets to conceive. A pregnancy is termed as a full term when it takes approx. 37 weeks. Even the babies who are born before this time are healthy and live a normal life. Most women go into preterm labor without really delivering their infants early.

**Chromosomal anomalies**

The possibility of chromosomal anomalies increases when two fetuses are involved. Non-identical fetuses have a higher chance of abnormalities. All the risks need to be evaluated in the third trimester and this will help the doctor to choose the type of labor. Development of abnormalities is not common in babies and depends upon the medical history and condition of the mother. Mothers who get pregnant after the age of 35 may have the higher chance of abnormalities. This all gets important for women considering genetic testing.

**Diabetes**

Diabetes is a common condition that is formed in the women who are expecting multiple babies. Although this condition is rare, but the doctor screen the mothers for this condition.

## Hypertension and preeclampsia

In the pregnancies where multiple fetuses are involved, there is a huge chance of hypertension. The number of embryos does not affect this condition. You will not see any physical signs of this ailment and women who are giving birth to twins are prone to this disease. Some women may also develop a condition known as preeclampsia. In this ailment, the woman may feel protein deficiency. The doctor will do some tests to make sure that the baby is not affected by this condition. More than forty percent woman who are expecting twins are affected by this disease.

## Intrauterine development limitation

This ailment of fetal development may affect more than fifteen percent pregnant women. The issue is significantly basic in triplets and in babies that offer a similar placenta. When the woman has a single placenta, there is a chance that one child gets more supplements from the mother's body than the other. There is no surety that which child will get preference, but this will cause an imbalance that can affect the health of the other child. Your doctor will analyze the condition of both the babies with the help of ultrasound.

## Twin-twin transfusion disorder

This condition is only limited to the babies who share the same placenta. When the babies have the same placenta, the veins are interconnected and this association may cause the blood imbalance in the babies. One baby might get more blood than the other and this may hinder the normal growth of the other baby. This can cause decreased development of the baby and this can cause premature birth as well. When this condition happens, the doctors prescribe some medications that ensure the normal growth of the baby.

**Multi-fetal pregnancy decrease**

Women who have multiple fetuses while they are pregnant may have an increased chance of delivering a healthy baby. Many researches also support this claim. When a woman is expecting more babies, the chance of premature delivery increases. The doctors will induce the richness treatment to make sure the multi-fetal pregnancies decrease and a healthy child is born. Many women ask the doctors to reduce their pregnancy to a singleton and this practice is getting common these days. Normally a maternal-fetal drug master plays out a multi-fetal pregnancy decrease somewhere in the range of 9 and 13 weeks in an exceptional focus. An experienced doctor can perform this procedure with ease and if the procedure is completed as per the right method, there is a very low risk involved. The doctor will walk you through all the possible solutions and ensure that you are ready to make the right choice. The doctors will perform the procedures after collecting data from your various tests and ensuring the delivery of a healthy baby.

**Selective termination**

A selective termination technique can be utilized in a multi-fetal pregnancy to end one of the babies when that embryo has a huge variation from the normal. A maternal-fetal prescription expert can play out this strategy if the embryos have separate placentas, with the goal that the medicine utilized can't traverse and influence the ordinary fetus. You need to take the help of a physician to ensure that the pregnancy is going on the right track.

## How to tackle premature birth of twins

When the uterus is expanded to a certain limit, this induces the process of labor. When you are pregnant with twins, the uterus will expand during the third trimester, and this can cause premature delivery. The dangers of premature delivery are increased when you have multiple fetuses in your body. As described earlier in this chapter, the average time taken for the birth of a single baby is forty weeks and it takes approximately 36 weeks for twins to conceive.

Doctors aren't sure what causes labor to begin in any pregnancy. Doctors are working on different approaches to avoid premature births in twin developments. Adding progesterone will help the doctors to shield the uterus and making sure that premature delivery is avoided. These practices will not completely safeguard the mother from premature delivery. The doctors try to find ways to highlight the issues in the women in the second trimester to prepare for premature delivery. You will need to visit doctor multiple times when you are having twins so that premature delivery can be stopped and the babies are born healthy. One way to tackle premature delivery is with the help of steroid shots. These steroids help the babies to develop the organs in a speedy fashion in case of a premature delivery.

The transvaginal ultrasound can be used to indicate early delivery in the women. The factors that are used to highlight early pregnancy are:

- Cervix Length: Before the labor, the cervix length will get shorter. In the week 16 to 24 of pregnancy, the cervical length is generally inspected. A medical officer will conduct these tests again to ensure that the safety of the children so you should be prepared for it.

- What is the width of cervix: Early enlargement is called funneling because that the cervix resembles a funnel on an ultrasound? The recurrence of the estimations relies upon your own individual situation; however, they're commonly taken about like clockwork. When the cervix has normal width and length, the chances of preterm labor are low. If the doctor feels that the cervix shape, length and width is abnormal, they will admit you to the emergency clinic.

Another test to foresee the probability of delivering early includes deciding the degree of fetal fibronectin. This substance in vaginal discharge is acquired by utilizing a unique swab. When there is a high risk of early pregnancy, the woman will have high fetal fibronectin levels. The doctor will surely give you some additional steroids for inducing the healthy growth of the baby if the fetal fibronectin test is positive. The time of labor and the position of the cervix does not affect the decision to give steroids.

# Planning another baby

It is the best thing to consult your doctor before you are planning to have another baby. The doctor will analyze your medical condition before you ought to get pregnant again. Presumably, the most significant thought is your general health. When a woman regains the lost supplements of the last pregnancy and is medically fit to have another child, the doctors to get pregnant again clear them. The time is different in different women and on average; it takes approx. 12 to 18 months for a woman to regain her normal condition. A recent study highlights that the woman who gets pregnant before this time may have some issues in the next pregnancy.

It is recommended that you should wait for having another baby until you are fully recovered from your last pregnancy. The women who had complications in the last pregnancy should not attempt to have another baby without consultation with the doctor. Many parents want some age gap between their children and you need to discuss with your partner. On the other hand, there are some couples who like to have kids who are of nearly the same age. The decision of the kids' age solely depends on you. It is advised that you consult with the doctor when about the perfect age gap between the children. Family medical history also plays an important part in fertilization so, ensure that you plan the kids before you are 35.

**Differentiating between each pregnancy**
You need to know that every pregnancy is unique and it is quite difficult to differentiate between pregnancies. A mother will

definitely have different experiences every time and she can differentiate in all the tiny details of pregnancy. The first pregnancy will have its fair share of problems. When you are pregnant for the second time, the complications will subside fairly. Regardless of what anyone tells you, recall your own first pregnancy experience and apply it on the second term of pregnancy to avoid any side-effect. Here is a list of some things that can help you differentiate between the first- and second-time pregnancy.

- When you are pregnant for the second time, the stomach muscles will be more relaxed. This condition is caused due to their stomach muscles have been extended by their last pregnancy and are currently relax. You will feel more bloated when you are pregnant again.
- There is a contraction in the nausea condition. Some women reported that nausea and fever were not severe in their second pregnancy, but we also have some cases that reported severe symptoms during the second pregnancy.
- You can easily identify earlier fetal movement.
- You will feel that the labor process is fairly simple when you are pregnant for the second time.
- The Braxton-hicks' compressions will be softer during the recurring pregnancies.
- Most women feel less anxious and restless in their second pregnancy.

Pregnancies may differ in many things but you will feel the same love for all the children that you have. You need to make sure that you follow the doctors recommendations and work on all the precaution to ensure a healthy baby.

In their third pregnancy, most women usually experience a unique sort of stress. There is nothing to be worried about. The stress will only make things worse for you. Some elevated stress when you are pregnant for the third time is fine but having tantrums will not help you in any way. If you are experiencing such feelings, trust us, you aren't the only one. Remember the odds of an issue aren't naturally more prominent in a third pregnancy, regardless of whether the initial two went easily.

**Giving birth after C-section**

When a woman give birth via the cesarean procedure, they usually ask if the woman will be able to give birth vaginally or not. Somewhat, the appropriate response relies upon which kind of cesarean you had before:

- **Low transverse**: One of the most used methods for cesarean delivery is low transverse. Women who give birth by this procedure can give birth via vaginal route. The danger of uterine burst is most reduced with this sort of entry point. As long as there are no complications in this procedure, the vaginal route can be used for the next delivery easily.

- **Classical**: in a classical style cesarean, the entry point is made at the top of the uterus. This type of cut can open any time and it is not safe for you to have a vaginal delivery after an old style cesarean delivery.

- **Low vertical**: A low-vertical cut is performed less as often as possible than a low-transverse entry point, but it enables the mother to endeavor to work and deliver in a resulting pregnancy.

The cut made on your skin doesn't mirror the kind of entry point on your uterus.

There was an old myth that the women who had cesarean delivery shall never give birth via vaginal route. They believed that this would tear open the old scar and can endanger the mother as well. In any case, studies have shown that the danger of such a burst is entirely low under 1 percent. Talk about the issues of the uterine burst with your doctor. A study showcases that more than seventy percent of women who gave via the cesarean process can deliver a healthy baby via the vagina. The success of the vaginal delivery after the cesarean solely depends on the type of procedure that you have gone through before. An experienced doctor will make sure that the babies are born healthy and you should leave the choice of procedure to the doctor. The choice of the medical professional and the clinic plays an important role in increasing the chance of the successful delivery. It would be best if you looked for the tips highlighted in the earlier section of the book to choose the right doctor for you.

For what reason would you need to deliver your next infant vaginally? The primary advantage is that in case you're effective, your recuperation is a lot shorter. There are many benefits of having a vaginal delivery. You will not have to go through a surgery to deliver a baby. You need to know that some vaginal deliveries will also have their fair share of problems. Different advantages of vaginal birth are as follows:

- You will not have to go through any surgery and will not have to face anesthetic issues.
- You will be free from infection
- It is possible to lose a lot of blood during the cesarean delivery and this is not the case with the vaginal delivery.

In all cases of pregnancy, there are some dangers and complications. Even recurring cesarean deliveries may have some complications so you need to be medically fit before you plan to get pregnant again.

**Belonging from a Non-traditional Family**

Single ladies and gay and lesbian couples bearing kids are turning out to be increasingly normal. You can be categorized as one of these classes, talking about your circumstance with your doctor is significant. Try not to stress that your doctor may pass judgment or is he/ she is going to mocking you. Doctors are prepared to be touchy to every one of patients' needs, and you're the same. Your professional seems to have an issue with your circumstance, proceed onward to somebody who's progressively under-standing the sooner, the better.

In many single parent and lesbian pregnancies, the dad of the infant isn't physically present. You need to make sure that you collect all the medical history and the family background with the doctor so they can help you during the pregnancy and identify any issue that may arise.

If the dad won't be around for the entire procedure, build your very own encouraging group of people. When you are a single parent, you need to make sure that you call a relative or sibling to be with you at this time. It would be best to have a partner when you are in the process of labor and pregnancy. It would be helpful in the process if this person also accompanies you during the visits to the doctor.

## How to prepare your children for newborn

Most parents anticipate having a second child explicitly because they need to give kin to the first. It is not necessary that the first child is prepared or want a sibling. You need to make sure that you understand the thinking of your child. You also need to understand the fact that the child may take some time to be friendly with the newborn. The accompanying segments offer a couple of thoughts regarding how to help set up the more seasoned one(s) for the fresh debut. Numerous medical clinics currently offer kin classes to enable your child to adapt. Contact the emergency clinic wherein you intend to deliver for data.

**Explaining Pregnancy**

The straightforwardness or trouble you may have presenting another child sister or sibling depends on a considerable amount on how old the senior kin is. Clarifying another infant to a 15-year-old is simple; on the other hand, telling the same process to a 15-month-old can be difficult. The ordeal will start when you have to tell the first child that you are pregnant. You will even face difficulty telling a 2-year-old that you are pregnant. The babies will not even understand if you are pregnant for some time. You do not need to tell the child right away that you are pregnant. They will probably not notice any change in you till the second and third trimester. It is sensible to tell the mature kids that you are pregnant as they can be very helpful in such scenarios. You can also take them to the ultrasound tests and they can also accompany you to the pre-birth visits. Kids can also help you buy things for the newborn and also help you select the name of the new child.

If the kid(s) will be sharing the same room or you will be changing the lodging of the kids, you need to let them know in advance. This change enables your older child to get an opportunity to adapt so she/he doesn't relate the new circumstance straightforwardly with the new infant's appearance. The kid(s) might be anxious when you are in the third trimester and cannot give proper attention to them. Do not get rattled if the kid(s) misbehave in any way. They might be thinking that your behavior will change when the newborn will come to the house and you need to sit with them and let them know this will not be the case. During this time, be steady and adoring. Remember your youngster for the arrangements however much as could be expected.

**Arrangement for babysitting during delivery**

It is obvious that your kids will be alone at home when you will go to the hospital for labor. You and your partner might need to stay in the hospital for the entire day. It is best that you find a babysitter for the kids that can take care of them while you are away. Planning is easy when you have an arranged delivery. Now you will probably understand why finding the due date is important. It helps you arrange these things in advance. It is difficult to pinpoint the exact time of delivery but it is good to be prepared for these types of things.

If you do not know about the time when you will conceive and need to stay in the hospital for some days, you need to book the babysitter in advance. It is wise to keep the kids at home when you are having a baby. When you are stable, you can meet your children as it safe for them to visit you in the medical center. When conceivable, telephone your kid at home while you're in the medical clinic to reveal to him/her that you're progressing nicely, particularly if your labor is curiously long. It is best to ask the doctor about the visiting hours and ask your partner to bring the children at these times. Having a new sibling will be botch interesting and fun for the kids and they might love to give present to the newborn. You need to take some gifts with you so that the kids can enjoy this time and give them to the newborn.

# Chapter 11:
# Breastfeeding

*You will learn*

---

*Why breastfeeding is essential*

*Getting into a breastfeeding routine*

---

Most women struggle hard to get the answer to a simple question that which type of milk is best for their baby either breast milk or formula milk? People will surely know the answer to this question. There are many advantages of breast milk. Mothers should always give breastmilk to their infants as it helps in stimulating the growth of the newborn babies. Breastmilk is known to have the perfect nutrients for newborns. The immune system of the baby that prevents and fights disease is boosted up with the help of antibodies that are present in the breast milk. Almost everyone knows the benefits of breast milk but there is the time when breastfeeding is impossible. In harsh times, feeding formula milk to your baby instead of breast milk shouldn't be your fault or make you guilty. Feelings of guilt and shame aren't good for you or your baby. You have to adjust to the situation and no mother can ever think anything bad for her baby.

The first few weeks for every new mother can be exhausting and demanding. You and your newborn baby both are facing a new reality and it needs some time to accommodate and adjust in the new phase of life. The phase of adjustment with the newborn baby is not only providing the baby with the required nourishment but in reality, it is the phase of making a bond of love with the baby. Through breast-feeing, you can feel the closeness and cuddling experience with your baby that help you in accepting the reality of being in a new relationship. Always try to find a calm and quiet place to feed your child where there are least chances of disturbance. Make this breastfeeding time memorable as soon your child will start feeding on his/her own.

## MAMMARY GLANDS

- Fat
- Lactiferous Duct
- Milk Pool / Lactiferous Sinus
- Loblue/Alveolus

**MOMMY'S ANGELS**
EDITORIAL STAFF
GROW YOUR TODDLER TO THE BEST

# Breast-Feeding and its Importance

Breast-feeding is equally beneficial for both the baby and the mother. It has a number of health benefits that last in the baby's body in his/her entire life. That is why mothers are encouraged to breast-feed their babies as long as required.

## The process of milk production

The production of milk during the period of breastfeeding is quite amazing. When you are about six months pregnant, the body will be ready to produce the breastmilk. At this time, colostrum (tiny droplets of yellowish liquid) may appear on the nipples of some women. The newborn baby will need increased protein in the first few days. The colostrum, which is filled with protein, will also help the newborn fight the infections. It doesn't contain lactose (milk sugar).

After 3-4 days of breastfeeding, milk supply gradually increases, and you may feel your breasts full and tender. Sometimes the breast may feel hard and lumpy when the glands are completely filled with milk. During the process of breastfeeding, milk-producing glands release milk which flows down to the milk ducts. Milk ducts are tiny openings that are located behind the dark circle of tissue that surrounds the nipple (areola). Baby's mouth works as a suction pump and compresses the areola, which forces the milk to pass out from the nipples. The sucking action of the baby completes the breastfeeding process.

Sucking action by the baby stimulates the nerve ending in your nipples. When the brain receives the message from the nerves, it releases oxytocin (a name of a hormone). Milk-producing glands in the breasts are affected by the oxytocin that results in ejaculating the milk to the feeding baby. This milk ejection process is also known as let-down reflex, may give you a tingling sensation. Your mammary glands will only be able to produce milk after the delivery of the baby. If you don't go for breast-feeding than the milk supplies your breasts will eventually stop. If you will breast-feed you, baby, your body will generate milk according to the demand. The more your breast is emptied, the more milk will be produced by the breasts. This all scenario of milk-production is based on demand and supply principle.

## Benefits for Mother

Breastfeeding will not only provide the required nutrients to newborn babies but also benefits mothers in a number of ways. The following are the few important benefits of breastfeeding for mothers.

### Delay in Periods

Breastfeeding plays an important role in extending the time between pregnancies. This is mainly because of the delay in monthly periods.

### Helps in faster recovery

Breastfeeding helps in faster recovery from childbirth. Oxytocin is released as a result of the baby's suction of breasts which helps in contracting the uterus. The hormone oxytocin recovers your uterus in the pre-pregnancy size more quickly after the delivery.

**Long-term Health Benefits**

Women may suffer from different kinds of cancers in the later stages of their lives. There are many long-term benefits of the breastfeeding as well. It protects the women from breast cancer as well. Other benefits of breastfeeding include the protection against uterine and ovarian cancer.

**Benefits for Baby**

The best thing which a newborn baby can get is his/her mother's milk. Breast-milk contains all the s and antibodies which an infant requires. The following are the benefits of breast-milk for a baby.

**Protection against disease**

According to a study, breast milk protects the baby from getting frequently sick. Breast milk contains antibodies that avoid childhood illness by building a strong immune system. The babies who are fed with breastmilk have fewer chances of disease such as ear infections, food allergies, and skin allergies. Apart from this, the babies will also be saved from colds and urinary tract infections.

Count of red blood cells (anemia) is also well maintained in breast-fed babies. Research suggests that breast milk may also protect the baby from sudden infant death syndrome (SIDS) also known as crib death. The risk of childhood leukemia is also slightly reduced in the breast-fed baby. A breastfed child is more protected against disease in his/her entire life. The chances of diabetes and heart stroke problems due to low cholesterol are greatly reduced due to breast milk.

**Complete Nutrition**

To fulfill the needs of your baby, you need the right amount of nutrients. There is no substitution of the breastmilk as all the nutrients are packed in it. It helps in the optimum growth of the newborn. Breast milk contains proteins, fats, carbohydrates, minerals and vitamins that are easy to digest and also helps in developing the brain and body of your baby. As your baby grows, the composition of breast milk changes according to the requirement of a breastfeeding baby.

**Protects a child from obesity**

According to studies on breast milk, breast-feeding provides protection to babies against obesity in their adulthood. Individuals who were breast-fed are less like to become fat in the later stages of their lives.

**Easy to digest**

. It is very easy to digest breastmilk. This is why it is given preference over the cow or packed milk. Breast milk remains in the baby's stomach for very less amount of time, which results in less gas and fewer constipation problems. Breast milk helps the baby's digestion system to function properly by killing some diarrhea-causing germs to avoid diarrhea problem

**Other major benefits**

Breastfeeding is an activity in which baby performs the sucking action to extract milk from the breasts. This particular activity helps in the development of your baby's facial muscles and jaws. The chances of getting a cavity at a later age are also greatly reduced through breastfeeding.

## Major Pros and Cons of Breast-feeding

There are some issues with the breastmilk that you also need to know. It is beneficial for the mother and baby but you also need to understand all the pros and cons of breastfeeding. Following are some factors that you need to consider when making this decision.

**Cost-saving:** Saving money may not be the top priority on your list when you have the child's benefit on your mind but choosing the breastmilk will help you to save money as you will not have to buy formula milk to feed the baby. You can also save money from buying bottles as you don't need them in breast-feeding.

**Helps in creating a bond:** With the help of breastfeeding, you can create a bond of closeness and intimacy between you and your newborn baby.

**Convenience:** Breastfeeding is easier than feeding the baby with bottle milk. Whenever the baby shows signs of hunger, he/she can be nourished anywhere and at any time with breast milk. In addition to this, no equipment for feeding is required and breast milk is also available all the time at the perfect temperature. Nighttime breast-feedings can be more convenient as you don't have to wake up for preparing the bottles of milk. You can simply feed your baby just by lying on his/her side.

**Perfect rest-intervals for mothers:** Breastfeeding time provides the perfect rest time for mothers as after every few hours your baby needs to be nourished.

The following are the few challenges that can be faced by mothers while doing breast-feeding.

**Sore Nipples:** During the breastfeeding phase, some women may face the problem of a breast infection or sore nipples. These problems are mainly caused due to improper positioning of breasts or applying inappropriate techniques of breast-feeding. To overcome such problems, you can take advice from a lactation consultant or consult with your primary health care provider and ask guidance about the proper positioning of breasts while feeding your baby.

**Exclusive feeding by mothers:** Early weeks of breastfeeding can be quite demanding for mothers. Baby needs to be nourished every two to three hours, day and night. This required physical effort can make mothers tired and even the father may feel left out. The partner can use the breast pump to store the milk for feeding the baby later. It may require a month to develop ample milk production, which can be extracted through a breast pump.

**Restrictions for mothers:** Mothers should have a proper diet when they are breastfeeding the child. Certain restrictions like alcohol are strictly prohibited for mothers because the alcohol can pass to the baby through breast milk. You also need to ensure that you do not use any medicine without consulting with the doctors. Some medications might get pass via breastmilk.

**Some physical side effects:** Hormones that are released during the process of breast-feeding may keep your vagina dry. This problem can be treated through using a water-based lubricating jelly. Establishing a regular pattern of your menstrual cycle may also take some time while breastfeeding.

## Situations when breast-feeding is not possible

Nature has given the ability of breast-feeding to almost every woman. Women's ability to breast-feed her baby doesn't depend upon the size of her breasts. Small breasts produce the same amount of milk as do the large breasts. Women who had undergone different kinds of breast surgeries like breast implants or breast reduction surgery are still capable of breast-feeding.

There can be some unfortunate situations when a woman is not allowed to breast-feed her baby and her doctor recommends to bottle-feed the baby. Your doctor can provide you suggestions about the best formula milk which can be given to your baby. Below are some worse situations, when mothers are not allowed to breast-feed the baby.

- You have been diagnosed with cancer and undergoing the treatment process.
- You indulge in alcohol. Alcohol or any other drugs you are taking can easily pass into your baby through breast milk.
- Infections like HIV, tuberculosis, hepatitis B or C or human T-cell lymph tropic virus can be transmitted through breast milk. If you are infected from any of these viruses, never breast-feed your baby.
- The effects of certain medication can pass into the baby through breast milk. If some medications can harm the baby, you need to make sure that you do not breastfeed for some time. These medications include blood pressure drugs, anti-anxiety drugs, anti-thyroid medications, and some sedatives. You need to be in constant communication with your doctor

and tell them about all the medications that you are using. They will tell you if you need to discontinue any medication.
- Any woman who has developed chickenpox (varicella) or West Nile virus should avoid breast-feeding her baby as such infections can transmit into the baby through breast milk. In this particular situation, your doctor can advise you better after analyzing your medical condition.
- When the newborn is suffering from certain health conditions such as galactosemia or phenylketonuria (PHU), the baby may require additional supplements to recover which can be provided through adapted formulas.
- Premature baby or the baby who isn't growing well require additional nutrients to overcome the problem of poor growth. In addition to breast milk, formula milk is advised to fulfill the needs of the baby who require additional nutrients.

**Vitamin D requirement**

Vitamin D is an essential vitamin for your newborn baby. If you partially or exclusively feed your baby with breast milk then consult with your doctor as breast milk doesn't contain enough vitamin D. Vitamin D helps in absorbing phosphorus and calcium which are essential vitamins for making strong bones. Lack of vitamin D can cause a disease known as rickets (weakening and softening of bones).

According to the Institute of Medicine and the American Academy of Pediatrics, 400 international units (IU) of vitamin D are required on a daily basis by an infant in its first year of life.

**Tips for your convenience**

It can be quite confusing if you are going to experience breastfeeding for the first time. This is normal behavior and many women had expressed the same feelings. Women whose breastfeeding goes right for the first time feels wonderful and accomplished. You need to stay calm in this situation. No doubt, breastfeeding is a natural process but many mothers don't know the right way of doing it because the activity of breastfeeding requires practice. Breastfeeding is a new skill for the mother as well as for the baby which means that this activity requires some time and practice before it goes perfectly well.

It is best that you breast feed the child when he/she is born. This is the perfect time according to many experts. If you cannot breastfeed the baby when they are born, consult with the doctor about the perfect time to do so. Outcomes of breast-feeding are greatly improved from early skin-to-skin contact. For better learning of your baby about breast-feeding, request the hospital nursing staff to avoid giving any bottles of water or formula milk to the baby unless advised by the doctor.

**Take advice when you require**

The birthing center or hospital is the best place to seek advice regarding breast-feeding. There is no shame in asking for help regarding breastfeeding. You can inquire about the right way to breast feed the child from the doctor or the nurse.

These experts can give you instructions and hints which can be helpful in nourishing your baby. After leaving the birthing center or hospital, you can arrange a knowledgeable infant feeding public health nurse to visit you for providing additional information about breast-feeding. Taking classes on breastfeeding is a good idea to enhance your knowledge and skills. For better nourishment of the baby, most birthing center and hospitals educate mothers through offering classes on effective feeding techniques.

**Additional supplies required**

Nursing bras provide additional support to lactating breasts. In nursing bras, the front of both cups can be opened which differentiate it from regular bras. This feature helps you to easily maneuver while holding your baby to perform the activity of breastfeeding.

Another important accessory that can help in breast-feeding is nursing pads. These pads are used to absorb the leaked milk from the breasts. They are placed between the breasts and the bra to soak all the leaked milk. They are slim in size and are disposable so many women wore them continuously.

**Don't feel panic**

You will make a strong bond with the child when you breastfeed him or her. Find a quiet and relaxing place to feed your baby. Place a glass of water or juice near to you as you may feel thirsty when your milk goes out from your body. Turn off your phone to avoid any interruption. You can also read a book or can watch the TV while breast-feeding your baby to get more relaxed. You need to stay relaxed when you are breastfeeding your child.

**Always breast-feed your baby in a comfortable position**

To get maximum relaxation, it is best for both of you to choose a comfortable position to perform breast-feeding. No matter where you are, either in a hospital chair, bed or lying on the bed. Putting a pillow behind your support. Sitting in a comfortable position should be your priority when you are breastfeeding your child. When sitting on a chair, try to have some support and always choose the chair with small arms.

**Baby feeding positions**

Breast-feeding starts by putting your baby in the right direction so that he/she can extract milk from the breasts easily. Hold your baby up and move your baby across your body in a way that his/her mouth touches your nipples. Make sure the whole body of your baby faces his/her head, back and hips are in a straight position. The other hand should be used to support the breast when breastfeeding the child. The weight of the breast should be supported by your hand and lightly squeeze your nipple to keep it in a straight forward direction. Different mothers have different breastfeeding positions and have their separate opinion about which position is more comforting. A few basic positions are described below so that you can choose one which fits you perfectly.

**Cradle Hold:** Cradle hold is one of the most common breast-feeding positions. You need to hold the baby in a comfortable position and place the head on your elbow. You can place a pillow to make it more comfortable for your baby. Your entire forearm will support the baby's head. To hold and support the breast, you can use your other free hand.

**Cross-Cradle Hold**: Adjust your baby in a position where the babyfaces your breast (tummy-to-tummy position). Hold the baby in the arm which is opposite to the breast from which you want to breast-feed. The open hand of the holding arm can be used to support the head of the baby. This allows you to get better control over the position of your baby. Use your other free hand to support the underside of the breast by making a U-shaped of the hand. This will help you to place your nipple in the baby's mouth.

**Clutch/Football Hold:** The elbow under the arm will be in a bent position and the hand of the arm will be providing support to the head of the baby. The face of your baby will be towards your breasts. For more convenience, you can place a pillow under your arm which will provide you ease and comfort. Sitting on an armchair with low positing arms can be a plus point. Use your free hand to support your feeding breast in a C-shaped position so that breasts can be aligned with the baby's mouth. In this position, the baby is not aligned with the tummy of the mother which is perfect for those mothers who are recovering from C-section. This feeding position is also popular among women with large breasts or women who are nursing small or premature babies.

**Side-lying Hold:** Sitting position is mostly advised to new mothers as it is the most convenient way of learning to breastfeed. After getting some expertise, many mothers prefer to breast-feed their babies while lying down. In this way, mothers can also relax their bodies. In the side-lying position, lay down on any of your sides either left or right, use your lower arm and hand to hold and keep the head of the baby near to your breast. Now use the upper arm and hand to grasp your breast and put it near the baby's lips.

## BREASTFEEDING POSITIONS

- CRADLE POSITION
- LYING DOWN
- FOOTBALL HOLD

MOMMY'S ANGELS
EDITORIAL STAFF
GROW YOUR TODDLER TO THE BEST!

**Breast-feeding to multiple babies**

When you have successfully established the ability to breastfeed, you can easily handle more than one baby. It is completely possible to cater to the breastfeeding needs of more than a single child. You can perform this by adopting a football (clutch) positioning method. Pillows can be used to support your arm and baby's head. It requires some creativity to breast-feed triplets. Two babies can be breastfed at a time and for the third baby, you can use a bottle. Again, the bottle can be used for the other baby at the next feeding. Your goal should be to provide breast milk to all the babies.

To get more information regarding an effective technique of breast-feeding, you can discuss your situation with your primary health care provider or can take advice from the lactation consultant. Ask them if they know any mother who undergone a similar situation and want to share any practical advice or can offer some support.

**Basics of Nursing**

When your baby doesn't immediately open his/her mouth to accept the breast, touch nipples on the face or cheek of your baby as a reaction, your baby will open mouth if he/she is hungry or interested in nursing. You need to put the baby's mouth on your breast as soon as he/she opens them. It is best to put the entire nipple in the baby's mouth. You should not get worried if the baby is not drinking milk. It will take some time for the baby to accept this norm. Expressing some milk on the baby's face can also encourage him/her to open mouth and latch on.

You may feel some surging sensation when the baby's mouth starts suckling your nipple. It is normal and after some suckling, that sensation of surging may disappear. If this particular sensation still exists, then sandwich your breast bit more tightly by gently pushing the head of the baby towards yourself. If this activity doesn't give you comfort, then stop the baby from breastfeeding by gently pushing it away from the breast but first remove the suction. When you want the baby to stop the suction, you need to gently put the finger on the side of the baby's mouth. Gently press the gums of the baby until the baby has stopped sucking the nipple. You may need to repeat this process until the baby stops sucking. After some time, you will be able to understand the breastfeeding process. With slow observations, you will get to know about the rhythmic movements that the child makes. This also helps you to know that the baby is swallowing the milk. You need to make sure that you do not block the baby's nose when you breastfeed the child. If you feel that the position is not comfortable for the bay, you need to change the position. You should not change the position if you feel that the baby is not showing any type of discomfort.

Both breasts should be offered to the baby for the purpose of feeding. It is necessary that you wait until the baby has proper fed from the first side and then change the side. When you change the side of the breast after equal time, it ensures the proper distribution of the milk.

The time of nursing mainly depends upon the need of your baby. Allow as much time as your baby desires to feed. It is best to change the breast when you are feeding the child. Normally it will take 30 minutes for a child to be fed. This is because the milk that comes first is known as foremilk which is protein-enriched and helpful in the growth of the baby. As the milk sucking process continues, the next phase of the milk starts coming which is known as hindmilk. Hindmilk contains fats and calories which helps the baby in gaining weight. Your baby will give you indications about when to change the side of your breast. So, wait for the signal of your baby before your switch sides of your breasts.

One of the best reasons of choosing the breast milk is that is easily digested by the baby. This is the main reason that the breastfed babies mostly show the signs of hunger after every few hours at first. New mothers often find this hectic to feed the babies all the time as they think that they are producing less milk and the baby remains hungry even after having a complete session of breastfeeding. The baby will grow at a steady pace when you breastfeed the baby and this will also give you the mental peace of mind and keep you safe from different diseases.

## Maintain your Health

Many new mothers forget to maintain their health and gives all attention and care to their newborn babies. It is a common phenomenon that the mothers will ignore their own health when they ought to take care of their babies. You need to make sure that you do not fall sick as this will also dampen the health of the child. As you need to breastfeed the child, you need to make sure that you take good care of your health. By following a few simple steps, you can maintain your health standards.

**Rest:** As a new mother, sometimes it seems really hard to get any rest. After you give birth to the baby, your body will be stripped from many vital vitamins and in order to regain your health, you need to make sure that you take proper rest. A good diet is also necessary in this stage. Milk-producing hormones are enhanced in the breasts after you have taken complete rest. Breastfeeding creates a soothing effect that can make you feel sleepy. So, try to complete your sleep according to the baby's sleeping schedule.

You can also take help from your younger children or from your partner to assist you in completing all the daily tasks. As a breastfeeding mother, never compromise on your rest or you can face health problems.

**Nutrition:** There are no food restrictions for breast-feeding mothers. If you are breast-feeding you, baby, try to eat a healthy and balanced diet. Mothers should take approximately 6-8 cups of fluid on a daily basis. Water, milk or juice can be used to fulfill the fluid requirement of your body.

Cooking on a daily basis can be difficult for new mothers. Snacks of healthy food items can be used to fulfill your food requirements. Your partner can also bring refreshments while you are nursing your baby.

## Tips for Breast Care

You might have to face some issues when you breastfeed the baby for the first time. When you are comfortable with this process, you will be able to tackle all the problems related to breastfeeding. Few are the common problems that can be experienced in breastfeeding.

**Fullness:** The breasts will feel full and tender after you give birth to the child. In this condition, it will be difficult for you to hold the nipples. The phenomenon of the swelling breast is known as engorgement. Due to this swelling, the milk will move slowly in the breasts. And this will also cause hindrance in the breastfeeding process. You can take some milk in your hand and feed the baby.

Although this solution is not permanent but it will help in easing the process. You can also support the breast with one hand. You need to place the hand on the areola and this will ensure a steady supply of breast milk. To get relief from engorgement, some women also get a warm shower to let-down some milk. A breast pump can also be used to express some milk out.

When some of your milk is released, you will definitely feel the softness in your areola and nipple. This eases the breast-feeding process and ensure a steady supply of milk to the baby. You can avoid the state of engorgement by having lengthy sessions of nursing to your baby. Try not to miss a feeding session and nurse your baby regularly. Continuous wearing of nursing bra throughout the day and night will be helpful in providing support to engorged breasts and provide you more comfort and ease in the days of breast-feeding.

An ice pack can be used to reduce breast swelling caused after nursing your baby. According to some mothers, breast tenderness can be relieved after having a warm shower. The engorgement will only last for some days after delivery and there is nothing to be worried about.

**Milk Ducts Blockage:** Milk ducts in the nipples are blocked sometimes, stopping the milk outflow. You can feel these blocked ducts through observing the hardness of the breasts or tender lumps. You need to make sure that you get this problem checked as the blockage can cause infection in the breasts. After breastfeeding the baby, if you still feel that some milk is left in the breast, use your hand or a breast pump to express the excess milk out. To relax the affected breast, you can also apply a warm compress or massage it before nursing your baby. If you are still facing the same problem after applying all the self-treatment procedure, then do consult with a lactation consultant or call your doctor to get better advice.

**Sore Nipples:** At the beginning, when the baby latches on, you may experience some discomfort in your nipples. This is common among breastfeeding mothers that are mainly caused due to cracked or tender nipples. Incorrect positioning and latching can cause sore nipples. Ensuring that the entire areola is in the baby's mouth can help prevent soreness. Make sure that the baby's head is in the right position when you are breast feeding. You need to make sure that baby's head is not in the free motion as it will put a lot of stress on the nipple and may cause soreness. Keeping the nipples moist will also help in preventing the soreness. You can use the milk to wet the nipples every time you breastfeed your child.

**Breast Infection:** The worst problem which can be faced by breast-feeding mothers is breast infection (mastitis). It is mainly caused when the mothers failed to empty the breast while breast-feeding. Germs can enter into your milk through the baby's mouth or from crack nipples. For babies, these germs are not harmful but they can infect you as they don't belong to your breast tissues.

You can diagnose mastitis infection through identifying its symptoms like fever, flu and body aches. After these symptoms, you can also face the problem of breast swelling, redness, and tenderness. If you develop any of these symptoms or sign, immediately consult with your doctor and he will definitely prescribe you some anti-biotic. Even with anti-biotic, you can keep nursing your baby as it will not harm your baby. Try to empty your breasts while feeding your baby to avoid clogged milk ducts. If you still feel pain in your breasts, use your hand to express some milk out from them while taking a warm shower.

**Other Methods of Pumping Your Breasts:**

You can use the breast pump to extract the milk from your nipples. This method can also be done with the hand. You need to understand that you cannot feed the baby all the time and storing the milk will help you a lot. In any case, most breastfeeding moms discover utilizing a breast pump simpler than manually expressing out milk.

There are different kinds of breast pumps that are available in the market. Testing out different breast pumps and selecting the right one is necessary. Breasts are a very sensitive area in a female's body, so you need to select the one which offers proper support and flexibility. If you're facing difficulty in making this choice, request help. Your primary care provider or a lactation consultant can assist you with settling on the best decision, and offer assistance and backing in case of any problem.

**How regularly will you utilize the breast pump?**

Manual pumps can be used to pump out the milk when you are going away for some time. It is not possible to be near the infant all the time. These pumps are small in size and are available at a modest rate. If you plan to go out for a couple of days or more, you will need to buy an electric pump and store the milk via this device. Electric pumps suck the breasts more successfully than do hand pump. This helps in extracting all milk from your breasts and keeps the milk supply secure.

### How quickly you need to pump?

A normal pumping session keeps going around 15 minutes a breast. The electric pump enables you to pump milk from both breasts. They take half time as compared to a single breast pump.

### How much does a breast pump cost?

There are many places where you can buy the breast pump. Many child stores, departmental stores and medical stores sell the breast pump. As far as the prices are concerned, you can purchase the manual breast pump for under fifty dollars. On the other hand, the electronic breast pumps cost an average of $200. They may have a milk carrying case as well. Having a breast pump is essential for you and this may help you to feed your baby when you are not near them. A few medical coverage plans cover the expense of leasing or purchasing a breast pump. Since there's a little danger of hygienic problems, it is recommended to purchase a brand breast pump for personal use. To avoid contamination and breast infection, never purchase a used breast pump for personal use.

### Is it easy to assemble and ship the breast pump?

The breast pump may be difficult to assemble and clean at the start but with some practice, you will be able to easily complete this task. You need to look for a lightweight model when you are trying to carry the breast pump with you at the office and other places. The breast pump is a small investment that can deem fruitful in the long run as well. Some breast pumps come with the carrying case as well and you can easily save the discarded milk in it. You also need to know that electric breast pumps cause some operational noise as well. You need to look for a model that has low noise.

**How can I adjust the suction?**

The same setting cannot be applicable for everyone as some feel comfortable in setting "A" while others feel comfortable at setting "B". This means that your breast pump should have to completely adjustable. Some pumps come with different suction levels. Ensure that you choose the model which comes with variable suction so that you can use it comfortably.

**What is the correct size of the breast shields?**

The shield is the cone-shaped cup on the top of the breast pump that needs to be placed on the breast when using. The suction cups come in different sizes. If you feel that the suction cup is small in size as compared to the breasts, you can check the manufacturers and buy another suction cup. If you are planning to use the pump on both breasts at the same time, look for the model that comes with two suction cups.

**How to Store Breast Milk**

You need to consult with the doctor about the dos and don'ts of storing breast milk. The breast milk needs to be stored perfectly to ensure its safety.

**To store breast milk, what kind of container is required?**

You need to make sure that the container or glass that you use to store the breast milk is thoroughly cleaned. All the foamy water should be discarded before you store the milk in it. You also need to heat the container as it will ensure the freshness of the milk. If you are planning to store the breastmilk for two to three days, you should use the plastic container. While efficient, plastic bags aren't prescribed for long haul breast milk storing since they may spill, release and become defiled more effectively than hard-sided containers. When using the milk in the plastic bag, you need to understand that certain components of the milk can stick to the plastic bag and this will deny the kid from having many vital vitamins.

**What's the ideal approach to store expressed bosom milk?**
Breast milk can be stored in the freezer. It is best to mark the breast milk so that it is not mixed with cow's milk. It is ideal to put the milk in the back of the freezer to ensure its freshness. Utilize your most fresh pumping first.

To limit waste, fill singular containers with the measure of milk your infant will require for one feeding. The breastmilk may expand when it is placed in the freezer so you can expect some spilling as well.

**Can I mix freshly expressed breast milk with stored milk?**
It is common to add fresh breast milk to the old milk that is stored in the freezer. Make sure that the old milk is not taken for four days and you need to take it out of the freezer for an hour before it can be mixed with the new milk. It is best to defrost the old milk to ensure both milks are easily mixed.

**For how many days can I keep expressed milk?**
The storing strategy is one thing that plays an important role in determining the time of which you can store the breast milk. Breast milk stored at room temperature can be safe to use for 4 to 8 hours.

If you are not planning to use the milk right away, it is advised that you store it in a freezer. The temperature of the freezer is one of the main factors that depend on how long the milk can be used safely. It is advised that you should not store the milk for more than three days in the freezer. You need to make sure that you use the milk as soon as possible. The milk contains many vital vitamins that will be lost if the milk is kept in the freezer for a long time.

Different examinations have appeared that refrigeration past two days may diminish the microscopic organisms killing properties of breast drain and long-haul freezer storage may bring down the nature of breast milk's lipids.

**How would I defrost frozen breast milk?**

It is best that you defrost the old milk first. When you are planning to use the defrosted milk, it is advised that you put the milk in the refrigerator the night before. You can also slowly warm the milk in the hot container. You need to make sure that the water does not interact with the mouth of the milk container. You should avoid defrosting the milk at room temperature. This increases the chance of the milk to get soiled.

These strategies can make an uneven appropriation of heat and damage the milk's antibodies. Utilize defrosted breast milk inside 24 hours. Dispose of any outstanding milk. Don't refreeze defrosted, or in part defrosted breast milk. It is perfectly normal for the child to drink the defrosted breast milk. The smell of the defrosted milk may be different from the freshly expressed milk.

**Is there anything else to know about breast milk storage?**

When you store the breast milk, it will form a lather on the top that will stick to the container as well. You need to mix the stored milk before feeding the baby, making sure that the foamy section is mixed with the milk completely. Always remember to gently shake the bottle.

**Continuing your routine work**

With a bit of arrangement and planning, you can perform both breast-feed and continue your routine work as well. A breast pump can be used for this purpose. You can continue your normal professional life after giving birth to the child. While some moms work from home, others have to go to the office and they cannot always take their babies with them. Due to this, storing the breast milk is best for the working women as the baby can get the vitamins at the right time and this will eliminate the hassle of feeding the baby from breasts every time. When you need to store a large quantity of milk, invest in the breast pump that has double suction cups. It will take just 15 minutes for the double breast pump to pump the milk. You can also use the breast pump at work and store the milk for later use. You can pump the milk at different times depending upon your routine. Keeping a difference in the time when you pump the milk helps a steady flow of milk and a decent supply.

**Bottle-feeding**

If you can't breast-feed or decide not to, you still have to make arrangements for your child to get complete nourishment. A wide variety of formula milk and cow milk options are available for the newborn. Most of them depend on dairy animals' milk. But be careful, never utilize normal dairy animals' milk as a substitute for formula. Even though dairy animals' milk is utilized as the establishment for a recipe, the milk has been changed drastically to make it alright for babies. It's dealt with appropriate heat to make the protein in it increasingly edible. More milk sugar (lactose) is added to make the focus like that of breast milk, and the fat (butterfat) is evacuated and supplanted with vegetable oils and creature fats that are all the more effectively processed by newborn children.

Baby formula contains the perfect measure of carbohydrates and the perfect percentage of fats and protein. The Food and Drug Administration screens the security of commercially manufactured newborn child formula. Every producer must test each group of formula to guarantee it has the necessary supplements and is free of contaminants.

Newborn child formula is prepared in the light of providing energy-based nourishment. The greater part of it contains calories that come from fat. A wide range of unsaturated fats makes up that fat. Those that go into newborn child recipes are explicitly chosen since they're like those found in breast milk. These unsaturated fats help in the advancement of your infant's mind and nervous system, just as in meeting his or her energy needs.

## Advantages and Disadvantages of Bottle-feeding

**Flexibility**: With the help of a bottle with formula, more than one person can feed the baby means anyone other than the mother can prepare and give the bottle to your baby. Hence, a few moms feel they have more freedom when they're bottle-feeding their babies. Bottle-feeding is also like by many partners as it permits them to put their share in the duties of feeding. Bottle-feeding can likewise exhibit a few difficulties, for example,

**Its preparation can be time-consuming:** Bottles must be arranged and warmed for each feeding. A steady supply of formula milk should be maintained by the parents. Nipples and bottles need to be washed properly to avoid contamination. If you go out on work or for an outing, you may need to take formula milk with you.

**Cost**: Most parents are concerned as formula milk is expensive and can upset their monthly budget.

**Baby acceptance of formula**: You have to try a few kinds of formula milk before selecting one for your newborn. As different formulas are suitable for different babies.

**Basics of Bottle-feeding:**

For the first time when you buy formula milk for your newborn, you may be surprised to see the number of options available in the market. Counsel your child's care supplier for advice about picking the correct formula. For most infants, an iron-sustained, cow's formula milk is the best decision.

A few exceptional formulae additionally are accessible, for example, those containing soy protein and protein hydrolysates. These recipes are made for explicit stomach related issues and ought to be utilized distinctly under the supervision of the health care provider. The iron-invigorated formula is significant for averting frailty and iron lack, which can cause slow improvement. Iron insufficiency isn't a chance in the initial, not many months of an infant's life. In any case, it can happen later in the first year. Iron lack in 6-to 10-month-old newborn children was previously iron supplementation.

Newborn child formula comes in three structures: powder, liquid concentrate, and ready-to-feed liquid. Both the powder and concentrate liquid formula must have an explicit measure of water added to them. Dry powder recipes, for the most part, are the most affordable.

If you choose to bottle-feed your infant with newborn child formula, you'll need the right supplies close by you when you bring your infant home from the medical clinic. Let the medicinal staff help you to introduce bottle-feeding to your newborn. The staff at the clinic or birthing center can give bottle-feeding equipment filled with formula during your recovery phase and tell you the best way to bottle-feed your infant. After that, you are all alone to bottle-feed your baby.

Equipment required for bottle-feeding regularly includes:

Four 4-ounce bottles (useful in the beginning)

Eight 8-ounce bottles (for intermediate level feeding)

Eight to 10 nipples, nipple rings, and nipple tops

A cup for measuring

A brush for bottle cleaning

Formula perfect for the baby feeding

Purchasing the correct equipment can be a difficult task for many new parents. You can take advice from the shopkeeper who is selling bottles for feeding or your read the manual given with the bottle. If you've never bottle-fed a child, taking a class will assist you with feeling progressively great when you bring your child home.

**How to start bottle-feeding:**

The bottles for feeding your child can be glass, plastic or plastic with a soft plastic liner. Bottles, for the most part, come in two sizes: 4 ounces and 8 ounces. The sum the bottle holds isn't a sign of how a lot your child needs to drink in a feeding. Your child may require less or more for some random nourishing.

Numerous kinds of nipples are available, which have openings measured to an infant's age. For some children, it has a little effect on which nipples you use. However, for a full-term child, don't choose excessively soft nipples structured for use by a premature child. A full-term infant should utilize an ordinary nipple. Utilize a similar sort of nipple for every one of the bottles.

It's significant that formula milk flows from the nipple at the right speed. Milk flow that is either excessively quick or too slow can make your infant swallow air, prompting stomach inconvenience and the requirement for visit burping. Test the progression of the nipple by flipping around the bottle and timing the drops. One drop for every second is about right. Nipples come in sizes for an infant, 3-month-old, half-year-old, etc., making the flow rate fitting for the infant's age.

## Preparing formula milk:

### Dairy animals' milk recipes:

Most newborn child formula is made with cow's milk that has been modified to look like breast milk. This gives the formula the correct equalization of nourishments and makes the formula simpler to process. Most children do well on cow's milk formula. In any case, a few infants, for example, those oversensitive to the proteins in cow's milk, need different kinds of newborn child formula.

### Soy-based recipes:

Soy-based newborn child formula might be a possibility for babies who are allergic or intolerable to cow's milk formula or to lactose, a sugar normally found in dairy animals' milk. A soy-based formula can likewise be valuable on the need to avoid creature proteins from your child's eating habits. In any case, babies who are hypersensitive to dairy animals' milk may likewise be adversely affected by soy milk.

### Protein hydrolysate recipes:

These are intended for babies who have a family history of milk or soy hypersensitivities. Protein hydrolysate formula is simpler to digest and more allergic to cause hypersensitive responses than are different sorts of formula. They are additionally called hypoallergenic formulas.

What's more, specific formulas are accessible for premature babies and babies who have certain medical conditions. Whatever type and types of formula you pick, exact preparation and refrigeration are basic, both to guarantee the fitting measure of sustenance furthermore, to defend the health of your infant.

Wash your hands before dealing with the formula or the equipment used to plan it. All equipment that you use to measure, blend and store formula should be washed with hot, clean water and afterward flushed and dried before each utilization.

Cleaning bottles and nipples aren't essential as long as you wash and flush them well. Utilize a bottle brush to wash bottles. Brush or rub the nipples completely to evacuate any remains of formula milk from the bottle. Wash well. You can likewise clean bottles also, nipples in the dishwasher.

In the case of utilizing powder formula or liquid concentrate formula, consistently include the precise measure of water advised in the instructions. Estimations on bottles might be off base, so pre-measure the water before adding it to the formula.

Utilizing excessively or too little water can be dangerous for your child. If the recipe is excessively weakened, your child won't get enough nourishment for their development needs also, to fulfill their hunger. A formula that is too concentrated puts pressure on the child's stomach, digestive system and kidneys, and could dry out your infant.

For the most part, you can store all readied recipes or liquid together in the fridge for as long as 48 hours. From that point onward, discard all unused recipe. Warming recipe isn't essential for healthful purposes; however, your infant may favor it warm. To warm recipe, set the bottle in warm water for a couple of moments.

Shake the bottle and test the temperature of the milk by dropping a couple of drops of formula on the highest point of your hand. Try not to microwave formula mils since this can cause traces of hot spots in the milk that can burn your child's mouth.

When you warm formula, don't refrigerate the remaining. Dispose of the unused remaining of the formula. It's ideal to make up formula when you need it, not progress of time. You may want to make up a bottle or two at night and store them in the refrigerator for using it at night times. This can help make evening time feedings simpler.

**Get into right position:**
The initial step to bottle-feeding is to make you and your infant in the right position. Locate a quiet place where you and your child won't be distracted. Support your infant in one arm, hold the bottle with the other and settle into a comfortable seat, ideally, one with low armrests. You may need to put a cushion on your lap under the child for help. Force your infant in toward you cozily however not very firmly, supported in your arm with their head and resting up in the curve of your elbow. This semi-upstanding position makes feeding a lot simpler.

Since you're prepared to begin feeding, help your infant prepare. Using the nipple of the bottle or a finger of the hand holding it, gently stroke your child's cheek close to the mouth. The touch will cause your infant to move in the direction of you, regularly with an opened mouth. At that point, contact the nipple to your child's lips or the edge of the mouth. Your child will open his or her mouth and will start sucking.

When feeding your child, position the bottle at around a 45-degree point. This edge keeps the nipple loaded with milk. Hold the bottle uplifted as your infant nourishes. Your child nods off while bottle-feeding, it might be because he or she has had enough milk, or gas has made your child full. Take the bottle away, burp your infant, and that point try to feed once more.

Continuously hold your infant while feeding. Never prop the bottle in the straight upward direction against your newborn baby. Propping may make your child upchuck and may prompt indulging.

# Chapter 12:
# Ten Important Points About Pregnancy

*You will learn*

---

*Concepts of the nine-month pregnancy*

*Fighting discomfort of pregnancy*

*Remembering your belly is not public property*

*What happens after delivery*

---

Try not to stress. We will not talk about any conspiracy that surrounds the pregnancy. You may have heard different nightmares of pregnancy from your sisters and cousins, but remember all that are myths. Pregnancy is a very fun and interesting time, and you need to enjoy it. Besides, different books frequently disregard this stuff, maybe in light of a legitimate concern for decency. All things considered, at the danger of being rude, we're going to offer it to you straight in this section.

**Pregnancy Lasts Longer than Nine Months**

Patients consistently ask, "How long along am I?" and we experience difficulty furnishing them an exact response. Pregnancy is said to most recent nine months; however, that number isn't actually exact. From the last menstrual period, the pregnancy lasts for 40 weeks or 280 days. (You think 40 weeks is quite a while? Simply be happy you're not an elephant, which has a growth time of 22 months!) When you are pregnant, you ought to be in the pregnancy phase for at least 10 months – calculating the time from when you know you are pregnant to delivering a healthy baby. On the schedule, be that as it may, most months contain a month in addition to a few days, so nine schedule months frequently contain near 40 weeks. Professionals talk as far as weeks when estimating gestational age since it's progressively exact and less befuddling.

**Others Can Drive You Crazy**

Companions, family members, associates, outsiders, and even your partner offer you spontaneous assessments and guidance and need to impart to you each pregnancy awfulness story they've at any point heard. They may disclose to you your back looks large, you're excessively fat (or excessively meager), or you shouldn't eat anything that you're placing in your mouth.

Wc understand these individuals, for the most part, have just honest goals when they disclose to you how their sister's pregnancy finished severely, or about the issue a companion of a companion had. They don't understand that they're expanding your tension. Try not to focus. Attempt to obligingly grin and overlook them.

**You Feel Exhausted in the First Trimester**

You might have to feel some weakness in the first trimester and this is because your body will be coming up with the changes in your body. You will also feel the urge to get additional sleep. Be it the workplace or the transit, and you will always be wanting to get some rest. You need to know that this weakness will go away and you will not feel tired in the second and third trimester. The tiredness will very off in the 13<sup>th</sup> week but you need to make sure you give proper rest to your body in the first three months of pregnancy. You will also feel the same tiredness when you are close to the labor process. Around week 30, the same feeling with engulfing you for a month.

**Round Ligament Pain Really Hurts**

The round tendons are located in the bottom part of the body and are located between the uterus and labia. When you are pregnant, the uterus will expand and this will cause the tendons to stretch. The pain is caused due to the stretchiness of the tendons. You will feel some pain in the crotch area between the 16 and 22 weeks of pregnancy. The pain that accompanies the stretchiness of the tendons will end, so there is no need to be worried about them. Changing the position regularly will also help in eliminating the pain. The pain will be completely gone by the 24 weeks.

**Your Belly Becomes a Hand Magnet**

After your stomach projects recognizably with pregnancy, you're probably going to discover all of a sudden everybody presumes contacting it is alright — not just your companions, relatives, and the individuals you work with, yet in addition the postal worker, the clerk at the store, and others you've never at any point met. Albeit a few ladies value the additional consideration, many think that it's an intrusion of privacy. You can either smile and bear it or find how to state, "Hello, uninvolved!"

## Hemorrhoids Are a Royal Pain in the Butt

Your closest companion may state she's enlightened you everything concerning her very own pregnancy. Due to the change in the shifting weights, you might feel some pain in the bottom section of the body. It is best to consult your doctor when you feel this pain. This pain will mostly be gone within fourteen days. In case you're lucky enough not to have them, understand how fortunate you are — and have compassion toward the various new moms who do have them.

## Now and then Women Poop While Pushing

Many patients ask about the solid discharge during the labor process. This is very common, and there is nothing to be ashamed of. The attendant will take care of any poop that occurs during the pregnancy. You and your partner do not have to worry about this as it is perfectly normal.

## The Weight Stays On after the Baby Comes Out

When the women give birth to the baby and the placenta, the woman will shed some weight. The woman may also have some swelling in the hands and feet which is completely normal. This additional water maintenance includes pounds. If you step on the scale immediately, you might be disillusioned at the number that surfaces. The expanding, for the most part, it takes about up to 14 days to leave.

## Medical clinic Pads are Relics from Your Mother's Era

At certain medical clinics, the attendants offer you sterile napkins from the 1920s — and a charming minimal versatile belt to hang them on. In case you're a time traveler or if for some other explanation you favor this sort, fantastic. You can also bring your home pads and containers for additional support.

## Breast Engorgement Really Sucks and Breast-encouraging Can Be a Production

When you deliver the baby, you might feel that your breasts become hard and big in size. The milk production also starts when the baby is delivered. We empower the entirety of our patients to bosom feed because of the advantages for the child; however, remember it might be more earnestly than you might suspect. Requiring some additional assistance and help is extremely regular. Luckily, most clinics have lactation masters that can assist you with draining the procedure along.

# Conclusion:

We are sure that after reading this book, you will understand all the pregnancy stages. Studying the book opens up new knowledge for you to analyze and will bring you ease regarding the pregnancy and its complications. All the complications and important sections of pregnancy are addressed adequately in this book.

We have compiled the sections in such a way that you get chronological information regarding pregnancy stages. From the day you know you are pregnant to the day you are going to give birth to the child, this book will provide real-time examples of any problem and their possible solutions.

The chapters of the book are devised in a manner that is easy to comprehend. We thank you for taking the time to read this book. You can provide feedback regarding this book as it will help us provide information in a useful and informative manner.

# The Postpartum Handbook

*The Deal with Depression, Sadness and New Mommy Issues*

**MOMMY'S ANGELS**
EDITORIAL STAFF
GROW YOUR TODDLER TO THE BEST!

# Chapter 1: Postpartum Introduction

Puerperium, also known as the postpartum period, refers to the time where the physiological changes that took place during pregnancy return to its non-pregnancy state after delivery.

The postpartum periods start right after childbirth. There is no exact timeframe for when this period ends, but it is estimated to last from 6 to 8 weeks after delivery. This is because almost all the effects of pregnancy have been returned to its pre-pregnancy state. However, the process in which all organs return to their original states is not the same for every woman and may take longer for some than for others.

There is a period where women are not fertile, and its duration depends on a number of factors, breastfeeding being one of them. This period is a variable, however, and even if the mother has not resumed menstruation, ovulation can still occur.

Many physiological and medical changes have taken place during this period so health-care providers should be aware of all the changes that women going through postpartum are undergoing and their own personal sensitivities and cultural differences that may involve restricting certain things and eating certain foods.

It is also common that women do not take part in sexual activity within several weeks of delivery.

# Physical Changes

Within a few hours or days of childbirth, you may begin to experience many changes in your body. These changes are typically normal and most of the time can be controlled with medication or exercise but it is not uncommon for there to be certain complications.

Here are some of the physical changes you are likely to go through:

**Breasts and Lactation**

Throughout pregnancy, your breasts will go through all the necessary changes to prepare for lactation, which is why they tend to grow in size during this time because of the hormone known as progesterone. After this, the endocrine system begins milk production. Within the first few days after childbirth, a fluid called colostrum starts to fill the breasts, which later turns into breast milk. Even though the breasts have grown in size during the pregnancy, they only become filled with colostrum after childbirth.

Women are usually asked to breastfeed immediately after delivery, to begin to develop a strong bond between mother and child.

When a baby begins to suck milk, a hormone called oxytocin will be released in your body. This hormone is responsible for contracting uterus, and this will prevent any bleeding. The sound of a baby crying can also release oxytocin.

It is also common to develop cracked nipples during the breastfeeding period, but this can be easily treated with medication.

You should receive all the necessary information regarding breastfeeding before childbirth, so that you don't have any difficulty later on, but don't hesitate to ask questions if you have them!

**Change to the Uterus**

The uterus is one of the organs that undergoes severe changes. This is because this organ, which weighs around one kilogram (2.2 pounds) is shrunken to almost 60 grams (0.14 pounds) containing only five milliliters of liquid. After delivery, the fundus of the uterus (which is the top part of the uterus) contracts to expel the placenta in a process takes around thirty minutes. This process is accompanied by a feeling of freezing, but it should feel dry, not wet.

At first, the smooth muscles of uterus contact and within 12 hours of birth, the uterus should be the level of the umbilicus (the navel). Within six weeks, the size of the uterus changes from one kilogram to 60-80 grams. Each day, the fundus contacts one centimeter down, toward the pelvic area. After two weeks, the uterus returns to its original place in the pelvic area, fully contracted.

The severity of the changes of uterine postpartum is longer and more intense in those women that have previously given birth to a child.

**Vagina, Cervix, and Perineum**

After childbirth, the vagina starts to return to its original size as it was before pregnancy and the cervix remains soft. For around six weeks of the postpartum period though, the vagina will keep discharging blood, mucus and other uterine tissue.

## Immune Response

During pregnancy, as the embryo grows, your immune responses are shut down. But when the postpartum period starts, the immune system reverts back to normal. This can result in infections that may have been previously present but never responded to by your body.

## Pain Control

It is very important that mothers-to-be receive information about what to expect in regards to pain. Depending on the person, getting this information can help to overcome the fear of what's to come.

After childbirth, perineal pain can have many negative effects on both mother and baby. These effects can also interfere with the care of the baby and can affect breastfeeding.

There can be pain in a few areas of your body, like uterine contractions, sore or cracked nipples or hemorrhoids. It is very important to give your doctor a detailed report on the type of pain so that they can prescribe medication or other remedies. Ice packs and a good hygiene can help in easing the pain, too.

There are also a variety of methods to control hemorrhoid pain. Here are some recommendations for managing the pain:

- Bath with warm water
- Hemorrhoid cream

- Drinking more fluids
- Lying down on your back
- Seitz baths

Uterine contractions are typically painful but this pain can be reduced by trying out different positions. Walking is known to be the best remedy for decreasing this type of pain. Since uterine contractions tend to be more painful during the breastfeeding period, medications are often recommended. In case of extreme pain, injections are preferred over oral medication.

The American Academy of Pediatrics recommends that an ongoing assessment should be performed after childbirth. For the first two hours, blood pressure, pulse, uterine position, and bleeding should be checked every 15 minutes. Body temperature should also be checked from time to time. This will protect you from many of the postpartum infections that can occur, especially puerperal sepsis, which is considered to be the main cause of maternal mortality.

**Changes in Nutrition**

Your caloric needs will also change after childbirth, depending on whether or not you chose to breastfeed your baby. A woman who isn't breastfeeding usually needs 1800-2000 kcal/day, while a breastfeeding mother needs 2300-2500 kcal/day. During the first 6 weeks of postpartum, calorie intake is increased by 333kcal/day and after six months it's around 400kcal/day.

Sometimes it is recommended that mothers use prescribed nutritional supplements, like iron and calcium. For other women though, it is more of a necessity than a recommendation, and they have to take prenatal vitamins. Fluid intake is also increased.

There are certain foods that aren't recommended if you're going for the breastfeeding option, since they may affect the baby. For instance, some doctors recommend that there should be no intake of caffeine, since it can cause fuzziness in the baby. Alcohol consumption is strongly dejected and greasy foods are also discouraged.

It is healthy to work toward regaining your weight prior to the pregnancy, but rapid weight loss can be detrimental to both the mother and the baby, and it reduces the supply of breastmilk. Eliminating carbohydrates or drastically increasing protein consumption as a weight loss method can also be harmful.

**Changes due to C-section**

If your baby was delivered through C-section, there are some additional points to keep in mind.

Before the C-section, it is very important that a urinary catheter is put in to prevent urinary retention. Additionally, the bedrest period recommended after a C-section tends to be longer than for natural birth. This is because the risk of blood clots is higher during surgery. To promote healthy blood circulation, leg exercises are highly recommended.

If you didn't plan for a C-section but had to have one, the hospital or clinic can provide counseling if this is a difficult process for you.

Some other physical changes that new mothers develop after childbirth are:

- Infections
- Difficulty urinating
- Constipation
- Hemorrhoids

Shivering- Around 25 to 30 percent of women can develop postpartum shivering. It usually starts around 1 hour post-delivery and lasts for 2 to 60 minutes after childbirth. The is no known cause for this, but there are a number of factors that can contribute to it, such as a drop in temperature after the strain of labor, bleeding, anesthesia or other drugs.

## Emotional Changes

Becoming a mother can be a very exciting adventure, but it is challenging as well. The changes you will experience are not limited to the physical aspect, but there will be emotional changes as well. The birth of a baby triggers many emotions in the mother that range from excitement to anxiety. Around the world, almost 80 percent of mothers experience "baby blues" or postpartum depression during the first couple of weeks after childbirth.

We will take a more in-depth look at emotional changes in following chapters.

# Chapter 2: Types of Postpartum

There are many misconceptions about the postpartum period. Many people believe that new mothers experience merely sadness, stress, or anxiety, aside from the physical changes. But the truth is that postpartum disorder has a variety wide of symptoms, and can actually be divided into many categories. Each of these has unique factors, symptoms, and treatment.

The way these disorders are categorized is based on the severity and duration of the symptoms. They are as follows:

- *Postpartum Blues (also known as baby blues)*
- *Postpartum Anxiety*
- *Postpartum Obsessive-Compulsive Disorder (OCD)*
- *Postpartum Bipolar Disorder*
- *Postpartum Panic Disorder*
- *Postpartum Psychosis*
- *Postpartum Post-Traumatic Stress Disorder*

## Postpartum Blues

Approximately 50% to 85% of women are affected by postpartum blues, making this the most common type of postpartum disorder. However, it is also the mildest of the disorders.

It typically starts within a week after delivery and can last anywhere from a few hours to a few days, and is usually gone after two weeks.

This disorder isn't just the one with the shortest duration, but its symptoms are also not as strong as the others. The symptoms don't affect the mother's daily routine and don't leave a heavy impact on her.

**Cause of postpartum blues**

There is no definitive cause for postpartum blues, but the hypothesis is that the psychological and physiological changes that occur after birth are the main reasons for it. Here are some of the contributing factors to postpartum blues:

- Fatigue after delivery
- Care of baby on a 24/7 schedule
- Lack of sleep
- Lack of support from family
- Marital strain
- Change in routines, either at home or at work
- Financial stress
- Social or cultural pressure
- Naive expectations of self
- Questioning ability to care for the baby
- Anger, loss or guilt

**Symptoms of postpartum blues**

The symptoms of postpartum blues usually vary from person to person, as well as from one pregnancy to next. In fact, many of its symptoms overlap with the normal symptoms that are experienced by new parents. Its symptoms include:

- Crying for no reason
- Irritability and anxiety
- Difficulty in making choices
- Mood swings and fatigue
- Loss of appetite and sleep
- Difficulty in concentration
- Negative symptoms intermingled with positive feelings

## **Prevention and treatment**

It is unclear whether taking preventative measures against postpartum blues is effective. However, knowing what to expect might be helpful in managing the symptoms. Since many people aren't aware of postpartum disorders, mothers suffering from them may feel an exacerbated sense of guilt at experiencing negative feelings during a time where they should be feeling joy and happiness. That's why it is of the utmost importance for parents to be aware of just how common these disorders are.

Although there's no real treatment for postpartum blues, since in the vast majority of cases the symptoms will disappear after two weeks, there are a number of recommendations to help ease the negative feelings.

- Reach out to your friends and family. Have a conversation with people you trust and share your feelings
- Maintain a well-balanced and healthy diet. After the birth of the baby, women can potentially neglect their diets in favor of caring for their child. Making sure that you eat healthy meals can go a long way in preventing mood swings

- Avoid alcohol and drug consumption
- Go outside and get some fresh air. Sometimes just going to a different place can help improve your mood
- Take some time to relax perform activities that you enjoy
- Ask for help. There is no shame in asking the people around you for help! Don't feel like you have to juggle everything on your own
- Ask other parents for advice
- Get deep, restorative sleep
- Don't expect perfection. Getting the hang of your new life with your baby will take time, so give yourself a chance to adjust. Way too many changes will be taking place around you, from healing your body, to adjusting your feeding and sleeping routines—cut yourself some slack!

If the symptoms remain after two weeks, it is recommended that you consult with your health-care professional. Be open and honest with your doctor and always follow up on your appointments.

## Postpartum Depression

While postpartum depression (PPD) may have some symptoms in common with postpartum blues, they are actually two different disorders with different treatments. Your doctor needs to be aware of all your symptoms in order to be able to give you the right diagnosis and, of course, the right treatment. That's why it's so important to be honest about your symptoms.

While over 80% experience baby blues, only 10-15% of women have been observed to develop postpartum depression.

Postpartum depression is linked to both emotional and physiological changes, although there is no clear link between chemical changes in the body and depression. During pregnancy, the levels of estrogen and progesterone in your body are increased extraordinarily and, only three days after childbirth, these levels drastically drop down to normal. This extreme change in hormonal levels is believed to be one of the causes for PPD.

PPD can last anywhere from a few days to several months after delivery. It is a mix of many complex feelings including anxiety, fear and sadness, and treatment is entirely dependent on the severity and duration of the symptoms.

Working with both your doctor and a psychiatrist will ensure the best outcome when it comes to treating PPD.

**Symptoms of Postpartum Depression**

Women with postpartum depression have described feeling restless, out of control, anxious, sad, overwhelmed, worried, etc.

Other symptoms include:

- Tiredness
- Irritability
- Feelings of hopelessness and isolation
- Increased or decreased appetite
- Insomnia or sleeping too much
- Feeling no connection with the baby
- Feeling unwilling to care for the baby
- Negative thoughts about yourself or the baby
- Thoughts of self-harm or harming the baby
- Crying for no apparent reason
- Difficulty in concentrating
- Trouble remembering things
- Apathy

- Unexplained pain
- Being unable to perform daily tasks
- Repeated thoughts that are uncontrollable
- Anxiety and panic attacks
- Feeling like you're a terrible mother

Postpartum depression is a real disorder that is exceedingly common, so don't think you're a bad mother or that you don't care about your child if you feel this way.

## **Early Warning Signs of Postpartum Depression**

When you have a baby, your productivity decreases and you cannot perform at your full potential. Not getting enough sleep is another big problem for new mothers.

Over ten percent of women are likely to suffer from PPD. If you are among these women, take some solace in knowing that you are not alone in the feelings of emptiness, sadness and exhaustion after giving birth. If you know what signs to look out for, you can seek the help you need at the earliest possible time and the sooner you seek treatment, the sooner you will get to live your normal life again.

### You Worry a Lot about Your Newborn

Every woman who just become a mother worries about the health of her child. When a woman faces premature birth, she is relatively more concerned about the overall health of the baby.

When you have given birth to a healthy baby but are still worrying a lot about the baby and are constantly thinking that you're going to be a bad mother, this might be the earliest sign of depression.

You Lose Interest in Things

After giving birth, you may begin to lose interest in your favorite activities, hobbies or interests. This feeling is normal for the first few days after childbirth, but if the feeling persists, it is a good idea to talk to your doctor about it. You need to tell your doctor about any changes in mood and habits. Timely consultation will help the doctor to analyze your condition and provide the best healthcare.

Changes in Your Sleep Pattern

It is obvious that your sleep patterns will drastically change when you have a baby. This is completely normal. But when your child is napping and you still feel restless, this means that your sleep patterns have changed. This leads to insomnia, which can lead to depression. Take note of your sleeping patterns after childbirth and report any anomalies to your doctor.

Stress

If you're picking fights with your partner or the people around you, feel like you're alone in raising your child and no one is helping you, and feel overwhelmed at everything you need to take care of, this is a sign of PPD.

Having Suicidal Thoughts

One of the advanced signs of postpartum depression are suicidal thoughts. You will find yourself thinking about harming yourself and/or your baby. You need to make sure that you seek immediate medical attention if you experience suicidal thoughts or thoughts of harming your baby.

Decision-Making Problems

Women usually feel tired after the birth of their child. This is one of the main reasons that you may not be able to make important decisions about your life. In some cases, you may even have trouble making the simplest decisions, like when to change the baby's diapers, when to take a shower, or when to take a nap. If you are facing difficulty in making these decisions, then it is possible that you are suffering from postpartum depression.

Baby Blues Do Not Get Better

It is evident that you will face some mood swings after the first two weeks of childbirth and that your condition will improve after this time. If you are not feeling better after two weeks, or you're feeling even worse, then you might be suffering from PPD.

Immense Sadness

It is normal to feel sad after you give birth to your baby. If the sadness and crying spells do not get better or you feel bad about becoming a parent, then you might be experiencing PPD.

History of Depression

This is not one of the strongest postpartum depression predictors but a woman who suffered from depression before she became pregnant is likely to develop postpartum depression. The feeling of emptiness after childbirth can be a trigger for past depression to return.

## Stressful Life Events

A death of a close relative or friend, or problems in your professional life may push you towards postpartum depression.

## Lack of Social Support

Coming back home after giving birth is a very special time. This is the time when you need your family and friends around you. Lack of social support is one of the factors that can trigger postpartum depression.

## Problems with your Partner

If you have a partner and your relationship is a difficult one, this can be one of the main factors that can cause postpartum.

If you're have problems with your partner, make sure that you both consult a couple's therapist.

## Self-Esteem Issues

A woman who has low self-esteem is likely to develop postpartum depression. Low self-esteem may also cause other psychological issues in the new mothers.

## Childcare Stress

A new mother will surely worry about the health and wellbeing of her baby. Some mothers take this stress to unmanageable levels though, and this additional stress may cause postpartum depression.

Unable to Understand Infant Issues

First-time mothers may not be able to easily understand their child's needs. This can cause them to feel anxious all the time, ultimately developing postpartum depression.

Being A Single Mother

Without a partner, raising a child is even more challenging and the stress of it all can lead to postpartum depression.

Unwanted Pregnancy

Postpartum depression can also occur because of unwanted or unplanned pregnancies. Women who become mothers at an early age are more likely to be affected.

Lower Socioeconomic Status

This mostly affects women living in developing countries where there are no proper healthcare facilities.

**Effects of Postpartum Depression on the Baby**

PPD is a serious illness that requires medical attention and can affect both the mother and the baby if not treated properly. If you're depressed, then your interactions with your baby will be strained, difficult and painful. This will prevent you from forming a strong, loving bond with your child. This lack of connection can affect the baby in the long-term, such as when expressing emotions, and they may even develop mental-health issues.

Babies are sensitive creatures, and they can not only sense, but also absorb their mother's mood. If you're sad, angry, scared or anxious all the time, this will also be reflected on your baby. This is why proper treatment is so important.

## **Treatment for Postpartum Depression**

Mental health professionals or health-care providers can help a mother suffering from a postpartum disorder. There are not lab tests that can be carried out to diagnose PPD, but there are other ways to diagnose it.

Counseling or therapy can be extremely helpful when suffering from PPD. You can call your insurance company to check what counseling services they cover.

Medication can also help in PPD. Even if you're breastfeeding, some antidepressants can be safely taken. You can also consult your mental health professional for this purpose and ask more about it.

## Postpartum Anxiety

Like postpartum depression, postpartum anxiety involves physical symptoms such as dizziness, rapid heart rate, nausea and the inability to concentrate. For some women, these symptoms start very early—normally, as soon as the baby is born—and can last up to a year. Approximately 20 to 35% of women suffer from postpartum anxiety.

Postpartum anxiety disorder is considered to be something of a hidden disorder, since only a few women recognize it as such and it goes undiagnosed for many. Since postpartum depression is much more commonly discussed than postpartum anxiety, it's easy for both mothers and medical professionals to mistake anxiety for PPD. Some feelings of anxiety also accompany PPD, which only adds to the complexity of making an accurate diagnosis. These two disorders usually go hand-in-hand, however, meaning that if a woman is suffering from postpartum depression, then she will also likely experience postpartum anxiety.

Even though postpartum anxiety isn't as widely discussed or studied as PPD, postpartum anxiety is actually the more common of the two to occur after giving birth. One study revealed that, out of 1024 women, 11% of women fell victim to postpartum anxiety, while only 7% suffered from postpartum depression.

**Causes of Postpartum Anxiety**

Anxiety is a normal reaction to protect both yourself and your child and most anxiety is adaptive. Most first-time parents can't help but having all sorts of terrible scenarios running through their heads about the horrible things that can to their baby—what if the fan falls on the baby, what if the baby slips and falls down the stairs, and so on.

This is a completely normal reaction, and a lot of parents having these thoughts can mostly ignore them, knowing that they're just background noise in their heads. However, anxiety is much more troublesome, and not as easy to deal with. It fills parents with a constant sense of dread and makes it impossible function properly.

The main reason for postpartum anxiety is, once again, the drastic drop of estrogen and progesterone levels in the body after childbirth. Additionally, all the massive life changes you're going through—bringing your baby home, your change in routine, responsibilities, sleep pattern, appetite, etc.—all contribute to postpartum anxiety.

## **Symptoms of Postpartum Anxiety**

- Constant fears and worries
- Extreme tension and stress
- Inability to relax
- Racing thoughts
- Fatigue, heart palpitation, and sweating
- Hyperventilation
- Nausea, vomiting and trembling of the body

## **Treatment of Postpartum Anxiety**

It's important to seek help if anxiety is causing sleep deprivation or if it is interfering with your daily routine. There are a number of treatments available for anxiety, but the first step is always to tell your symptoms to your doctor.

Depending on the severity, talk therapy can be a great treatment for anxiety. A therapist or psychologist with experience in treating postpartum anxiety will give you the necessary tools to deal with this disorder. In more extreme cases, medication may be prescribed temporarily.

## Postpartum Obsessive-Compulsive Disorder (OCD)

Postpartum Obsessive-Compulsive Disorder is different from regular OCD in that it is solely focused on the mother's thoughts and behaviors towards their newborn.

It is not uncommon for pregnant women to experience an array of emotions after the arrival of a new baby. Postpartum OCD, however, is characterized by recurrent thoughts and behaviors that are in response to a perceived danger. These thoughts are so invasive that they disturb your daily routine. Women suffering from this disorder are aware of their thoughts, but don't know how to manage and control these symptoms.

There are plenty of treatments available now for postpartum OCD and women do not have to suffer from it anymore.

**Causes of Postpartum OCD**

There is currently no known cause for this disorder. Its onset seems to be directly related to the mother's mental health history. The biochemical changes in the body after the birth of the baby, along with the chronic fatigue and worries that accompany having a baby, can lead to the development of postpartum OCD.

Many women who suffered from OCD before getting pregnant found that their symptoms increased after the birth of their baby.

It is also important to know that the biological causes of postpartum OCD in women are not the same as those for men.

## **Symptoms of Postpartum OCD**

A grouping of obsessions and compulsions are included in the symptoms of OCD. Here are some of the symptoms of common obsessions:

- *Unwanted thoughts of hurting the baby such as dropping or throwing him*
- *Concerns about accidentally causing the baby harm*
- *Obtrusive thoughts of suffocating the baby*
- *Annoying feelings of sexually molesting the baby*
- *Fear of making poor decisions that will harm the baby*
- *Fear that the baby will suffer from serious disease*
- *Fear of exposing the baby to toxins and other chemicals*


Given below are some of the symptoms of common compulsions:

- *Getting rid of sharp objects such as knives*
- *Not feeding the baby out of fear of poisoning them*
- *Not changing the baby's diaper out fear of sexually abusing them*
- *Avoid watching TV or reading news that involves child abuse*
- *Asking reassurance from family members that child has not been harmed*
- *Obsessively checking the baby why they're asleep*

## Treatment of Postpartum OCD

The treatment for postpartum OCD usually involves medication and therapy. Cognitive-behavioral therapy and psychotherapy help work through the feelings and thoughts in a safe environment.

Psychiatrists also suggest a course of medication such as antidepressants that will help to overcome compulsions and obsessions. Anti-anxiety medications like benzodiazepine is also effective in providing relief.

# Postpartum Bipolar Disorder

Research shows that approximately 21% to 54% of women who suffer from PPD can potentially develop postpartum bipolar disorder.

Screening for postpartum bipolar disorder should happen in the first three months after childbirth in order to get an accurate diagnosis. Inadequate screening, lack of awareness of this disorder and hypomanic symptoms that can be mistaken for the joy of having a child all contribute to postpartum bipolar disorder.

## Causes of Bipolar Disorder

Potential triggers for postpartum bipolar disorder are premature birth, cesarean delivery, gestational hypertension and antepartum hemorrhage.

Maternal PPD has long-term effects on a child's life but, bipolar disorder has no long-term effects. Being younger, unplanned pregnancy and depression are all factors of bipolar disorder.

## **Symptoms of Postpartum Bipolar Disorder**

Starting with depression, a patient of bipolar disorder also shows many other symptoms as:

- Feelings of euphoria
- Grandiose self-image
- High irritability and agitation
- Decreased desire to sleep
- Racing thoughts
- Impulsive behavior
- Feelings of hopelessness
- Suicidal thoughts
- Self-harm

Almost 17% of women with bipolar disorder have thoughts of self-harm. In the first postpartum year, the suicidal prevalence was almost 6.2%.

## **Treatment of Postpartum Bipolar Disorder**

It is crucial to get professional help for postpartum bipolar disorder as soon as possible. It's even more important to get an accurate diagnosis for this disorder because there are certain antidepressants that can induce mania in bipolar patients.

There are some mood stabilizers, like valproate, that are safe for new mothers to use even if they're breastfeeding. If the depression continues even with the mood stabilizer, your physician will have to recommend an antidepressant that is safe to use and doesn't induce manic episodes.

Because of the complexity of this disorder, and the possible side effects of many of the drugs used to control it, it is of vital importance that you give constant updates to your doctor so that the proper alterations can be made to medication and doses.

## Postpartum Panic Disorder

Unlike postpartum depression, postpartum panic disorder is a condition that triggers worry and fears instead of depression.

Postpartum panic disorder can sometimes be extremely crippling and damaging to women's health. It is actually a type of postpartum anxiety disorder that damages mental health and interferes with daily functioning. The anxious thoughts common in anxiety disorder can become full-blown panic attacks.

Any anxious thought can become the trigger for a panic attack, but postpartum panic attacks are usually linked to worries concerning your baby.

Approximately 4 to 10% of mothers develop postpartum panic disorder. Often, this disorder goes undiagnosed and untreated, partly because mothers may choose to ignore the symptoms and try to fight through them, or because it is misdiagnosed as simple anxiety.

This is why it's important for new mothers to be aware that panic disorder goes much further than just being worried. Panic attacks can cause serious mental and physical issues and tend to interfere severely with everyday life.

**Causes of Postpartum Panic Disorder**

To a certain degree, any type of postpartum disorder is due to the sudden change in hormones. However, there are many different factors that can contribute to developing postpartum panic disorder. Different bodies have their own natural response to fear and anxiety and, in some cases, when this fear becomes high, the body experiences a panic attack. If the panic attacks become frequent, then this is an indicator of panic disorder. Additionally, women with a history of the following may also be at risk of getting this disorder:

- Past history of anxiety
- Previous diagnosis of a panic attack
- Thyroid dysfunction
- Childhood trauma
- Fatigue and/or insomnia

## Symptoms of Panic Disorder

Symptoms for this disorder can start after two days of childbirth and can last up to almost 12 months. Given below are signs and symptoms of women suffering from postpartum panic disorder:

- Difficulty concentrating or remembering things

- Difficulty in completing tasks
- Easily distracted
- Indecisiveness and inability to relax
- Insomnia, fatigue, and loss of appetite
- Feeling uneasy for a long period of time
- Agitation and irritability
- Overwhelming and excessive anxiety
- Avoiding things out of fear or worry
- Agoraphobia (fear of being in public or open spaces)
- Suicidal thoughts or attempts
- Panic attacks

Here are three distinct but commons fears that women with postpartum panic disorder usually experience:

- Fear of death
- Fear of lost control
- Fear of going mad

## **Treatment of Postpartum Panic Disorder**

There are various treatments for postpartum panic disorder but the first step is to learn to recognize the symptoms and communicate them to a mental health professional.

Selective Serotonin Reuptake Inhibitors (SSRIs) are a type of antidepressant that can help in treating postpartum panic disorder. They can take several weeks to start working however, so some physicians may prescribe other antidepressant such as benzodiazepines in the meantime.

With the combination of both medication and therapy, women suffering from postpartum panic disorder can achieve full recovery.

## Postpartum Psychosis

Within the first three weeks after childbirth can experience a more severe level of mental illness. This can include auditory and/or visual hallucinations—hearing or seeing things that aren't there—and/or delusions—strong belief in irrational things. Auditory hallucinations are more common than visual hallucinations.

Other symptoms include confusion and disorientation, excessive energy and agitation, paranoia, obsessive thoughts about your baby, attempts to self-harm or harm the baby or insomnia.

Women suffering from this disorder should be treated properly and medical attention should be provided to in order to avoid any harm coming to them or the baby.

### Symptoms of Postpartum Psychosis

If you experience the following symptoms, visit your physician or mental health professional:

- Unable to sleep
- Unable to think clearly
- Hallucinations or delusions
- Obsessive and fearful thoughts about the baby
- Suspicion of other people
- Paranoia
- Loss of appetite

- Thoughts of hurting yourself or the baby

**Causes of Postpartum Psychosis**

Aside from hormonal changes, cultural, environmental and biological factors can also contribute to developing postpartum psychosis. Lack of sleep also plays a role. Factors that increase women's risk for postpartum psychosis are:

- History of bipolar disorder
- History of postpartum psychosis in a previous pregnancy
- Family history of postpartum psychosis
- History of schizophrenia
- Termination of psychiatric medication for pregnancy

## Treatment of Postpartum Psychosis

Postpartum psychosis is a medical emergency and you should immediately call 911 or other emergency services, or have someone who can take you to the emergency room.

Treatment of psychotic episodes include:

- Antipsychotics: They reduce hallucinations and delusions. Examples include risperidone, ziprasidone, and aripiprazole, etc.
- Mood stabilizers: Manic episodes are reduced by mood stabilizers. Examples include lithium, lamotrigine, etc.
- Electroconvulsive therapy is very effective for women who do not respond to medication. A controlled amount of electromagnetic stimulation is given to the brain, which "resets" the disturbances caused by psychosis.

# Postpartum Post-Traumatic Stress Disorder

PTSD is generally considered an anxiety disorder, but it relates more specifically to trauma and stress. PTSD affects approximately 10% of women, but this percentage is increased during the postpartum period, affecting around 12.7% of women after childbirth and 13.6% up to 6 months afterwards.

## **Causes of Postpartum PTSD**

There's very little information on postpartum PTSD, which means this disorder often goes underdiagnosed and undertreated. Potential trauma that can cause postpartum PTSD includes:

- Unexpected C-section
- Use of vacuum extractors or pincers for delivering the baby
- Feelings of helplessness and lack of support during childbirth

Women who experienced severe physical difficulty or injury related to the pregnancy or childbirth—postpartum hemorrhage, unexpected hysterectomy, perineal trauma or cardiac disease—as well as women who experienced trauma in the past such as rape or sexual abuse are at higher risk of getting postpartum PTSD.

Feelings of isolation, infertility, and abortion or miscarriage can also lead to postpartum PTSD.

Anxiety occurring late in the pregnancy is also a predictor for PTSD. If a newborn has to spend time in NICU (neonatal intensive care unit), then the likelihood of postpartum PTSD becomes much more extreme.

## Symptoms of postpartum PTSD

The symptoms of PTSD can last for several months and include the following:

- Difficulty recalling a traumatic past event (which in this case may be the birth of your baby)
- Nervousness and panic attacks
- Irritability
- Insomnia
- Flashbacks or hallucinations
- Avoiding thoughts, feelings, places or events associated with a traumatic event

## Treatment of Postpartum PTSD

It's important your physician and/or healthcare providers to play a preventive role for PTSD patients. With appropriate sleep, nutrition, and exercise, PTSD symptoms can be reduced.

PTSD is treatable with both therapy and medication. SSRIs can be very helpful for PTSD patients.

Therapy for PTSD is different from that of postpartum depression since techniques for re-framing and re-processing are more commonly used in treating PTSD. In this kind of therapy, the patient is taken back to the traumatic memory, positive elements are re-framed, stories from their birth are told and then the patient is returned to the present to assess the effect of their trauma on their bodies, minds and emotions.

If you have a partner, involving them in your therapeutic process can have excellent results.

# Chapter 3: How to Overcome Negative Thoughts

It's very easy to let yourself be completely overcome by your negative thoughts. Most of us spend the vast majority of our time inside our own head, focusing on the unsatisfactory aspects of our lives or worrying about our future. Our emotions have a very strong grip over our thoughts. They have the power to make our thoughts difficult to deal with and not easy to let go of. It's quite common that negative thoughts rob us of our happiness, leaving us with worries and distracting us from our goals.

Our minds work in such a way that they can cleverly convince us of things that aren't true, things that aren't happening, or things that will never happen. These false thoughts reinforce our negative feelings, which is why it's important to stop and take a moment to recognize which thoughts are real and which are made up.

The following are some types of thought distortions that contribute to negative thoughts:

<u>Black-and-White Thinking</u>

Black-and-white thinking means only seeing things either one way or another, there is no in-between them. A situation is either fantastic, or absolutely terrible and questions only have a yes or no answer.

Personalizing

This involves assuming all the blame for someone else's bad mood. When someone doesn't smile when they see you, for instance, then it must mean that you've done something wrong. In personalization, you are constantly finding faults in yourself and making yourself responsible for every bad situation that occurs around you.

Filter Thinking

When someone is filter thinking, they will only focus on the negative aspect of any given situation. Finding the positive side to anything becomes impossible.

Catastrophizing

Catastrophizing is when you start thinking that the absolute worst is going to happen, which can make a bad situation even worse.

## **Controlling Your Negative Thoughts**

Controlling our negative thoughts is a struggle in itself, but it's not impossible. Yoga and meditation are great ways to let go of negative thoughts and can help you to stay in the present moment. With continuous practice, you can learn to control your negative thoughts and can spend your life freely and happily. Negative patterns are replaced with good habits and behaviors that actually help you and this can make a huge difference in your life.

When it comes to the postpartum period, you can learn to control your negative thoughts using the following techniques:

**Challenge Negative Thoughts**

Whenever a negative thought comes into your mind, don't just accept it as the truth—try to think clearly about whether it's true or not.

A good technique for this is imagining that a close friend is going through the situation that triggered the bad thought. Imagine your friend telling you all about it and then try to think of what you say to them, what you would recommend they do and how you would help them. Now apply this same logic on yourself and try to find a logical way out of a problem. Don't assume that the worst will happen and don't blame yourself for being in that situation.

**Question Your Thoughts**

Self-talk is another great technique for questioning your negative thoughts. Self-talk is like a running commentary about your thoughts, a voice inside your head that examines, challenges and questions the thoughts that come into your head.

However, since you are the moderator of your self-talk, it is also likely that you can exaggerate the importance or veracity of your negative thoughts even when trying to question them.

Here are some of ways in which you could potentially sabotage your self-talk:

*Focusing on the Negative*

This is essentially the same as thought filtering where we only focus on our negative thoughts and leave out everything positive. For example, a new mother may start thinking that they're going to be a terrible parent and that their baby will never love then. The reality is that you're probably going through a postpartum disorder, and things really aren't as bad as you're imagining them to be.

*"Should"*

Sometimes we set limitations on ourselves based on how we "should" act or things that "should" happen. For example, a postpartum mother may set a deadline for herself that within three days after childbirth, her child "should" develop an attachment to her. But we are only setting ourselves up for failure by setting deadline like this, since the mother is likely to become depressed or anxious if what she planned for doesn't happen as it "should".

*Overgeneralizing*

This means taking one example of a situation or one previous experience and believing it to be true for everything that will happen in the future. For example, if a baby cries uncontrollably when their mother picks them up for the first time, then the mother might think that the baby will always cry when she picks them up again.

*All-or-Nothing Thinking*

All-or-nothing thinking is the same as black and white thinking. For example, mothers with PPD will believe that if they can't get rid of their depression now then they will be stuck with it for the rest of their lives.

**Take a Break from Negative Thoughts**

If you feel that a negative thought is starting to consume too much of your time and energy, try taking a step back from the situation and taking a break from it. Do things that distract you from your thoughts for a while.

**Choose Your Thoughts**

You can control your negative thoughts by picking and choosing what thoughts you allow to remain in your head. This is easier said than done, but there are some simple techniques that you can apply to help you with this.

One such technique is to keep a journal where you can write down your thoughts. Externalizing thoughts that were previously just in your head can help you get some perspective and you may naturally come to the conclusion that you shouldn't keep investing your energy on one negative thought.

By repeating this process every day—or as often as you can—you will slowly start to sift through your negative thoughts and find all the positive things you can focus on instead.

**Don't Judge Yourself**

It's very important not to judge yourself if you're having negative thoughts. More often than not, they're the result of one of the postpartum disorders, and not your fault at all. Having negative thoughts doesn't make you a bad mother or a bad person. The very first step in overcoming these difficult times is to know that you are not at fault for your thoughts and not to judge yourself.

**Practice gratitude**

Research has shown time and again that practicing gratitude for the positive things in your life can have an amazing and wonderful impact in your state of mind. Even in the most trying of times, there will always be something to be grateful for.

Set aside some time at the end of your day to sit down and think about the good things in your life. Even if you only find one thing, that is fine. Take the time to be sincerely grateful for it.

Another good technique is to write down the things you're grateful for in pieces of paper and using them to fill a jar. Whenever you're feeling down, take one of the slips of paper out of the jar and read it.

**Focus on your strength**

Always focus on your strengths instead of focusing on your weaknesses. It's human nature always be aware of the negative aspects of ourselves, but by choosing to focus on your virtues, you will slowly be able to control your negative thoughts.

Try finding your strength by thinking of your baby. It's true that you may be experiencing hard times due to a postpartum disorder, but if you focus on being strong so you can take care of your baby, you may be able to find strength within yourself that you didn't know you had.

**Talk about it**

Talk therapy is known to be very effective for women who are suffering from postpartum depression. When you are having negative thoughts, talking about it can help to overcome it.

**Go for a short workout**

Exercise is vitally important for new mothers, but especially so if they're suffering postpartum depression. Even a short workout can go a long way in helping to overcome negative thoughts and fighting anxiety. This is because exercise boosts the production of BDNF (brain-developed neurotrophic factor), a protein that helps the brain to perform its functions in a more effective way.

Additionally, exercise releases endorphins, known as the feel-good hormone, which helps boost your emotional wellbeing.

Yet another perk of working out is that you will start to feel more confident after even a short workout. Increased feelings of confidence and a boosted self-esteem will help you to deal with the negative situations around you.

**Get more social contact**

When you engage in social activity, it's a given that you will have less time to entertain your negative thoughts. Moreover, by being socially active you will be able to see the lives of other people and will absorb some of that positive energy.

## Coping in a healthy way

It's very important for you to perform activities that bring positive things to your life and environment. Don't resort to drug or alcohol as a way of coping to cope with your negative thoughts.

## Don't blame yourself

The very first thing you need to do if you want to be able to control your negative thoughts is to stop blaming yourself.

Blaming yourself only makes the process of overcoming your negative thoughts much harder, since you keep thinking about the situation and get stuck in that circle of negativity.

Having a postpartum disorder is not your fault, you didn't do anything to deserve having it, and it's something that can happen to any new mother. It does not make you a bad mother and you need to understand this as soon as possible.

## Release your thoughts and keep them moving along

When you want to get rid of your negative thoughts, you might start to push these thoughts away from your mind. But fighting your negative thoughts takes way too much time and energy, and in the end, it only makes a bad situation even worse.

The best approach to get rid of your negative thoughts is not pushing them out it but accepting that they are a part of your life right now and learning to live with them.

There are plenty of meditation techniques that can help you learn to acknowledge your thoughts and then patiently letting them go their way without fighting them.

## Understanding Your Concerns and Releasing Negative Thoughts

Another day dawns and you are not feeling any affection towards your baby. A flood of negative thoughts will pass through your mind. You need to remember two things.

First, you need to understand your concerns that are causing a lack of control.

Second, you need to acknowledge your thoughts and patiently ask them to leave your mind.

Don't think that just because you haven't fixed the problem yet, you will never be able to. Likewise, don't hang tightly onto each thought that comes into your mind. Learning to let them go will make these thoughts lose their influence on you.

Letting go of your thoughts instead of pushing them out will take a huge weight off your shoulders and will make you feel more relaxed and keep your mind open for many different thoughts. If you have a long-lasting habit of negative thinking then it may take some time to develop roots of positive thoughts.

Get some fresh air

An open atmosphere and fresh air are great to relax your mind. When you surround yourself with nature you will automatically start to feel much better—let nature energize you and bring positive thoughts to your mind.

Get into some activity

It is said that an idle mind brings only negativity—you will feel and think about every little thing over and over. Your mind will be filled with negativity if you don't get involved in any activity after the birth of your baby. This is because you will spend an inordinate amount of time in your own head, which only makes problems seem bigger than they are.

It's very important for you to get involved in any activity that you enjoy so that you can keep your mind busy and not let the negative thoughts in.

Do some yoga

We all know by now about the benefits of yoga. It can help you meditate as you exercise your body and is a great way to get some control over negative thoughts and develop a positive attitude.

A lot of women practice yoga during their pregnancy, but it is equally important to continue doing it even after the baby is born.

Seek professional help

When dealing with postpartum disorders and negative thoughts, it's always best to seek professional help. The World Health Organization is now providing mental health professionals to help women deal with these types of problems. One of the best types of therapy for dealing with negative thoughts Cognitive-Behavioral Therapy (CBT).

Cognitive-Behavioral Therapy

CBT is actually a kind of talk therapy that helps you to overcome your problems by changing your way of thinking. It helps you change your outlook on life to make it into a positive one. It is used for treating anxiety whether in anxiety patients and works really well with women experiencing postpartum disorders too.

**How it works:**

CBT is a kind of therapy that is entirely based on your thoughts. It handles problem-solving in a very positive way, starting by breaking one big problem into smaller parts. You are then shown how these smaller problems can be solved by changing negative patterns in your thoughts and behavior in order to improve you general wellbeing.

CBT has nothing to do with your past, it just focuses on your current situation. It also employs many practical techniques to improve your state of mind.

This therapy works in sessions where you have to meet your therapist every other week to keep them informed of your present state. Its treatment requires anywhere from 5 to 20 sessions.

# Tips to overcome negative thoughts at home

*1. If you find yourself in what appears to be a negative circumstance, locate something positive or supportive.*

If you've had a difficulty, your outlook may start to turn depressing and this gives way to negative thoughts.

*2. News flash: People think about you way less than you think they do.*

It's very easy to fall into the trap of thinking that the people around you will criticize the things you do or fail to accomplish. This way of thinking will make you constantly question your choices and even keep you from doing things that may be right for you.

The truth is however, that people don't really think about you as much as you think they do. Everyone has their hands full with their own problems, their children, occupations, pets, pastimes and feelings of dread and stress (like for instance what other people think of *them*).

If you acknowledge this fact and liberate yourself from the weight of what other people think about you, you will be able to finally redirect your energy and attention to the things in your life that really count.

*3. Question your thoughts*

Again, always question your negative thoughts.

If thought taps you on the shoulder and attempts to develop in your brain, you have to scrutinize it. Don't get excessively centered on one little misstep or one terrible day. Rather, focus on the other aspects of your life.

The closer you look at your bad thoughts, the easier it will be to realize that because you did one thing incorrectly, it doesn't mean everything you do is wrong. One negative thing doesn't mean that things will deteriorate and remain that way forever.

Developing this questioning nature will help to ground you in reality and give you some perspective.

*4. Eliminate the cynicism from your environment.*

What you let into your brain in your day-to-day existence will a tremendous impact on you. So be very selective in what you let in.

If this is challenging for you, start little by little. Pinpoint activities and people that bring joy and light into your life and focus on these. Do your best to avoid or outright eliminate sources of stress and bad feelings.

*5. Quit making mountains out of molehills.*

To prevent a little negative idea from turning into a major beast in your brain, stand up to it early on. You can do that by using tip #3 right now.

Or you can add a little perspective. Do this by asking yourself things like: Will this be an issue in 5 years? Or even 5 weeks?

This answer is likely that it won't, and that you were just beginning to make a mountain out of a molehill.

*6. Talk it over.*

Suppressing negative thoughts that are clouding your entire psyche won't help. So let them out. Talk about the circumstances or your thoughts with somebody close to you. Venting for a while can frequently help you with seeing the circumstance in a new light. Additionally, you will be able to obtain the point of view from an outside source, and you can also get some help in figuring out how to handle the problem.

*7. Live in and return to this minute.*

When you're in the middle of a negative thought, you're always either thinking about something that has already happened, or something that has not happened yet.

To shake yourself out of this, return your attention completely to this minute. Into what's here, in the present moment. Start to make it a habit to focus on the now and you'll soon be able to get rid of your negative thoughts in favor of more pleasant ones.

Give yourself a moment right now to take some deep breaths. Make sure you're breathing in through your nose. Let the air fill you all the way down to your abdomen. Then, let it out again through your nose. During this time, focus exclusively on the air filling your lungs, and how your body feels.

Do this as many times as you want. Then, take a look at your surroundings.

Enjoy this brief reprieve, escape your head, and put your consideration on what's around you at this moment. Nothing else. Center on the individuals strolling outside your window, the muted words and commotions from the road, the scents around you, the sun shining on your skin or the night cooling it down.

*8. Try not to let the dubious feelings of dread drag you down.*

One basic error people make regarding their fears is to get frightened and run away from them instead of looking more closely at them.

It's normal to feel that trepidation and to need to maintain a strategic distance from your fears. But keeping your distance will keep you from truly knowing just how terrible a situation really is, and you may end up making it out to be way worse.

So ask yourself this: What's the most terrible that could happen right now?

The moment you face a fear head on, with your feet solidly planted on the ground, then you frequently understand that the most terrible that could happen isn't actually that awful.

By doing this, you gain clarity about a bad circumstance and what you can realistically do about it to lessen its effect on your life.

*9. Bring positive energy into another person's life.*

If you find that you're still caught up in negative thinking, you can take a break from being in your own head and focus your energy outwards to another person. A couple of approaches to bring inspiration to somebody's life are:

Be caring. Offer kind words, hold open a door for someone, offer your seat on public transportation, etc.

Be helpful. Offer people guidance and advice that has worked for you in the past.

Be there. Focus on what the other person is saying and really listen.

*10. Start the day in a way that sets a positive mood for the rest of your day.*

A critical or negative beginning to your day makes it difficult to keep a positive attitude. If you start off with a cheerier outlook, your day is much more likely to go better than you thought, and you will be able to ward off the bad thoughts much more easily.

# Chapter 4: Doctor's Help

When we talk about treatment for postpartum disorders, the first person you have to think about is your doctor. It's vitally important that you consult your doctor as soon as you start to experience any symptoms of a postpartum disorder. This is because the more you delay your treatment, the stronger the symptoms can get.

It is also important to know how to talk to your doctor about your symptoms and what to expect in return. The first course of action that your doctor may recommend for treating a postpartum disorder is therapy.

Next, your doctor may recommend one of two types of treatments:

- Pharmacological treatment
- Non-pharmacological treatment

## Pharmacological treatment

### Antidepressants

Postpartum depression can be thought of as a variant of depression and antidepressant medication responds similarly to both. Antidepressants cause a metabolic change in the postpartum period. The antidepressant your doctor prescribes to you will vary based on many factors, such as your level of distress or your medical history.

While research is still scarce, so far there are four types of antidepressants for the treatment of PPD.

*Fluoxetine or fluoxetine plus CBT*

One study on the effect of fluoxetine showed that women receiving both fluoxetine and therapy (in this case, CBT), and women receiving just fluoxetine were significantly the same. The baseline of depressive symptoms among the women in this study was very mild though and findings cannot be easily generalized if the population had more severe symptoms of depression. Women who were breastfeeding were excluded from this study.

*Paroxetine or paroxetine plus CBT*

In another study, 35 women were divided into two groups: one group was asked to take paroxetine, while the second group was given paroxetine plus CBT for 12 weeks. The response rate for the paroxetine group was 87.5% and the combined group was 78.9%, with both the groups showing significant improvement in depressive symptoms.

*Paroxetine or Placebo*

Thirty-one women participated in this study and were divided into two groups: 17 were given paroxetine and 14 were given a placebo over the course of 8 weeks. After the trial, researchers found a lower severity score and a high remission rate.

*Nortriptyline and sertraline*

There are very few studies that run a trial using two different types of medication. In this particular study, it was shown that nortriptyline and sertraline gave almost similar outcomes. After 8 weeks of treatment, both groups showed similar response rates and remission rates. Response rates were: nortriptyline 69% and sertraline 56%; and remission rates were: nortriptyline 48% and sertraline 46%. The side effect profile was different in both groups but the side effect burden was the same. Both groups were equivalent and showed improvement.

Many other medications are effective for the treatment of postpartum such as:

- Sertraline
- Venlafaxine
- Nefazodone
- Fluvoxamine
- Bupropion

These studies were sponsored by pharmaceutical companies and were conducted on a very small group including 13 to 14 participants. Though there was a little comparison of medications to placebo, all the data taken from these studies showed that medication helps a lot in treating depression and these antidepressants are very effective for treating postpartum depression in particular.

Some experts have suggested that if the patient has taken an antidepressant in the past, then that's the first one that should be considered when treating PPD.

Two placebo-controlled studies

Two placebo-controlled studies have been taken into consideration for treating PPD. In one study, sertraline was given to non-depressed women in minimum quantities immediately after the birth of their baby and it prevented recurrence and prolonged relapse time.

In another study, the patients received nortriptyline and no difference was found in recurrence and relapse time. Research is still needed to conclude whether antidepressants that are given after childbirth can prevent PPD or not.

## Breastfeeding Considerations

The benefits of breastfeeding have been described many organizations, including the World Health Organization. Doctors recommend that a baby should be breastfed for at least for 6 months. The potential effects that antidepressants have on breastfeeding are of greater concern to every mother and physician. Young infants are very vulnerable to these drugs, since their renal and circulatory systems are not yet fully developed.

Experts recommend non-pharmacological treatment for mothers that are nursing a young baby.

Although there is not enough data on medication for mothers who are breastfeeding, it is known that sertraline and paroxetine are the least detectable in infant plasma and citalopram and fluoxetine are highly excreted by breastfeeding.

Rather than focusing on what medication a mother should take, the baby's pediatrician should be aware of the baby's exposure to everything and should monitor any and all changes with the baby, whether it's feeding patterns or sleeping patterns.

## Non-Pharmacological Treatment
### *Psychotherapy*

We have already discussed that psychotherapy is considered to be the most effective way of treating postpartum disorders. If you come across people who have suffered from this, then the first advice that they will give to you is that you should consult a therapist. So, who is a psychotherapist, exactly? To clarify it, different types of psychotherapies are given below:

*Interpersonal Psychotherapy*

*Cognitive-Behavioral Therapy*

*Dialectical Behavioral Therapy*

*Psychodynamic Psychotherapy*

*Eye Movement Desensitization and Reprocessing*

*Solution-Focused Brief Psychotherapy*

*Group Therapy*

*Couples Therapy*

**Interpersonal Psychotherapy**

Interpersonal therapy only lasts for about 12 to 16 weeks and is considered to be the most effective type of therapy. An IPT therapist is very active and straight-forward in the therapeutic process and its main goal is to give relief. IPT is actually built on the evidence that postpartum is present in four problem areas that are:

Grief: Acknowledging the loss that occurs within yourself, any change in your relationships and/or any other loss.

Role Transitions: The life change transitions that make you lose your independence and social transitions that cause a change in social networks.

Interpersonal disputes: Disputes that start after the birth of a child, whether intimacy with your partner or having unmet expectations.

Interpersonal Deficits: The struggle that you are going through for your relationship, which can cause distress.

IPT is manual-based therapy and it is teaching many communication skills that will build confidence in you and will give you social support.

## Cognitive-Behavioral Therapy

CBT is known to be very efficient in treating postpartum OCD. CBT actually works with the concept that the way you feel depends on the way you think. So, this therapy helps mothers to control their thoughts. A CBT therapist will help you identify your automatic thoughts, evaluate them and become aware that these thoughts are not helpful. Therapists will help you explore and change your underlying beliefs, helps to differentiate between real and false threats and helps in developing more helpful perspectives.

CBT will help you to develop strategies to manage stress. For stopping irrational thoughts, CBT uses different tools such as exposure therapy, homework, shopping thoughts and so on. Mindfulness-Based Cognitive Therapy is also a form of therapy that helps in mindfulness meditation.

## Dialectical Behavioral Therapy

DBT was basically a treatment for Borderline Personality Disorder but now it's being used for many disorders, such as anxiety. Homework and practices are both used as part of the DBT process. DBT is an effective treatment for the following categories:

*Mindfulness*

*Distress tolerance*

*Emotional regulation*

*Interpersonal effectiveness*

Individual and group therapies support DBT. It gives you a specific guideline for teaching those skills that specifically reduces distress.

## Psychodynamic Psychotherapy

One of the earliest types of psychotherapy is psychodynamic psychotherapy, that focuses on the past to understand the present. Psychodynamic therapists believe that our present distress has a very strong relationship with our bad childhood and when we become able to identify these thoughts, we will become able to deal with them and will be less tangled in our past.

This therapy looks into the early experiences that have played a part in forming beliefs about yourself and makes you realize that these thoughts are not helpful. As a mother working with a psychodynamic therapist, you will talk about your relationship with your parents and other people so that your unconscious way of thinking can be uncovered. This approach is thought to be very important because, in order for there to be change, there needs to be understanding first.

## Eye Movement Desensitization and Reprocessing

EMDR is known to be a very effective treatment for trauma and because of this it is being used for treating postpartum PTSD too. This therapy requires a specific type of training. EMDR along with its specific technique for reducing the effects of trauma also uses both CBT and psychodynamic therapy. Traumatic experiences are stored in either the right or left side of the brain. The right side is emotional and feeling-based and the left side is logical and intellectual. EMDR used bilateral stimulation—either eye-movement or bilateral sound—to reprocess the memories that are being used for body awareness. EMDR helps mothers to develop a sense of thought that is positive and healing.

## Solution-Focused Brief Psychotherapy

Solution-focused brief psychotherapy focuses on the specific problem and finds a solution for it. Unlike other therapies, it does not depend on any past or traumatic experiences. It stands away from the past and just focuses on the mother's present strength and skills. A lot of this therapy is just focused on finding the solution rather than problem-solving. This therapy requires many sessions for beneficial treatment but as it does not focus on the root of the problem, mental health experts believe that this therapy is not long-lasting.

## Group Therapy

Group therapy involves the support of the community. Many psychotherapists facilitate creating a true group therapy session. It helps group members to identify their thoughts and solve their personal disputes. A postpartum depression support group uses psycho-education that includes the mother's disorder, its causes, possible treatments, life strategies for wellness and so on.

The goal of the PPD support group is to help mothers to be heard, to show them that they are not alone, to make them talk about their struggles and worries.

## Couples Therapy

The aim goal of couple's therapy is to provide a safe space for a couple when their relationship is not at a good place. In this setting, the couple is asked to address their negative patterns and are made to talk and listen to each other. In couple's therapy, couples address their conflict, issues that are causing conflicts and individual needs for maintaining a healthy relationship.

When you are interviewing new therapists, it's appropriate to ask which therapy they have practiced in the past. Different therapists use different types of therapies in their work. A therapist who has a very specific training can use any type of therapy for a mother who is dealing with postpartum disorders.

**How you should talk to your doctor about postpartum**

Given below are some ways experts suggest that you talk to your doctor about postpartum depression.

First, you need to choose the doctor that gives you the most comfort. It doesn't matter if they're a pediatrician or a family doctor. Select a doctor you can trust, and who is more likely to pay attention to your concerns. It can be very difficult to open up and share your feelings with a doctor. But the longer you take to share your feelings, the longer it will take for you to start getting better. As soon as you feel uncomfortable about anything, let your doctor know instantly.

Gather as much information as you can about PPD. Learn about it so that you may have all the information about your problem and can ask as many questions as you can from your doctor. Be very specific about your feelings and don't feel afraid to talk about them. Write down all of your symptoms and your questions on a piece of paper so that when you visit your doctor you don't forget anything. And If you have any previous history of anxiety or depression, be sure to share that experience with the doctor.

If you have any fears about talking about your feelings, let your doctor know about them too. These are just reflections of your personality; it is not your fault, so don't feel bad about it because it does not make you a bad mother.

Do not let your fear overcome you, and don't stop from saying what you need to say. As mentioned before, don't pay too much attention to what people may think of you for getting help.

If you have any physical symptoms, get a thorough check-up of your thyroid and whatever blood work your doctor recommends.

If the doctor recommends any antidepressants, feel free to ask anything you want about the medication. Do not hesitate to ask anything because it is your right to know. This is all about your body and you have to know about everything before taking the medication.

Makes sure that you follow up on your appointments. If you are breastfeeding, your doctors need to know about that because medication will be different for mothers who breastfeed their children, and there are some medications that are excreted through breastmilk. Make sure to inform your doctor about every possibility because it's not only about you but it is also for your baby.

If at any time you feel that you are not being properly treated or not taken seriously, you need to seriously consider changing your doctor. Ask for a referral to a doctor who treats postpartum women specifically. You do not have to hesitate or feel shy about it. It's your right to look for a doctor who treats you the best way possible.

You can ask for help from anyone, either your family or friends, and can see things from other perspectives too. In this way, you can double-check information that will later help you.

Always remember it's hard to advocate for your own health when you are feeling bad but it's for your own good and you need to do it. It is your right to have a doctor that is supportive and well-informed about your all issues.

# Chapter 5: Postpartum in Fathers

Postpartum in fathers is a very common phenomenon. Approximately 2 to 25% of fathers are affected by their partner's pregnancy. According to the American Academy of Pediatrics, if the mother has postpartum depression too, then this percentage can increase up to 50%. It can prove to be very dangerous for the whole family, especially the children.

According to recent studies, it is proved that for having postpartum depression, it is not necessary that you give birth to the child. Studies have suggested that the ratio of postpartum depression in fathers is approximately 7 to 10%, and fathers are more likely to spank their children.

The University of Southern California has studied the link between depression and sagging testosterone in fathers. They also argued that postpartum is not just for women but is also found in new dads. These studies have found that as high testosterone level in fathers helps against depression, it increases the risk of depression in mothers.

We know that testosterone level drops in fathers and they get postpartum depression but what we don't know is the reason for this.

Parents who adopt also seem to develop PPD, but the reasons for this are as yet unknown.

A hypothetical case

Mr. M, a 35-year-old father, went to his physician because he was not sleeping. He reports that after the birth of his baby, he only sleeps 4 hours a day and gets up before the expected time. Due to this reason, he is feeling low energy in his body. He reports that he exhausted, that he does not find pleasure in any activity, whether it's playing any game or just watching television. He also reports that he is being very rude to his co-workers and family and is not finding any interest in his work anymore. He feels guilty for treating his family this way and was also questioning himself for becoming a father. Mr. M also reports a depressed mood "on and off" in his early 20s but it was never treated. Various tests were performed but there were no abnormalities.

## Fathers' Experience After Birth

Some mental health experts question whether or not fathers really experience PPD after their the birth of their child. But a great many studies show that the postpartum period is one of the hardest times for both men and women. New parents are never fully prepared for all the major changes that will occur in your life after the birth of your child. Additionally, fathers are given instructions on how to care for their partner if she is suffering from a postpartum disorder but rarely tell them how to take care of themselves.

We know that the hormonal changes in women after childbirth are massive, but similarly, fathers also go through many hormonal changes. The depression between father and mother is like apples and oranges.

## Hormonal Changes in Fathers

It is believed that men don't go through any hormonal changes because they are not giving birth to the baby. However, fathers also experience hormonal changes after childbirth.

It is clear that testosterone levels drop in fathers. One idea for why this happens is that if is a lower testosterone level, then the father will be less aggressive and more caring. But it is not just testosterone levels that change in fathers, but many other hormones like estradiol and prolactin also change as it changes in women. So, hormones also play a vital role in having postpartum depression in new fathers.

## Neural and Behavioral Changes in Fathers

Researchers are now exploring hormonal, neural and behavioral changes in new fathers. They are conducting different trials on fathers, one of which consists in giving them vasopressin nasally and looking at its effects.

Yes, fathers who have their first babies do go through some neural changes. The anterior cingulate cortex, paracingulate gyrus and supplemental areas of the brain become much more active when the father hears the crying of their baby. MRI scanning is done to check these changes

Similarly, when the father holds his baby for the first time and touches their soft skin and develops physical contact with them, his behavior also changes. His emotions change at that time and he develops a sense of love towards the baby. Suddenly, his whole personality changes and he becomes more caring and protective.

## Symptoms of Postpartum in Fathers

The kind of depression that men and women experience is very different from one another. These are some of the symptoms that fathers experience in postpartum:

- Increased anger
- Increased use of alcohol or drugs
- Frustration or bad temper
- Fierce behavior
- Noteworthy weight gain or weight loss
- Isolation from friends or family
- Very easily stressed
- Irresponsibility or risk-taking (this behavior can include extra-marital relationship or agitation)
- Feelings of discouragement
- Increase in complaints about many physical problems such as headache or pain in any other body part
- Concentration or inspiration problems
- No interest in activities like work or sex
- Concerns about productivity at work or school
- Fatigue

- Crying for no reason
- Angry about their feelings and expectations of fatherhood
- Recurrent thoughts of suicide or death

## Factors affecting fathers in postpartum

There are many factors that affect fathers when their partner gives birth to their baby. These factors are responsible for their depression. The factors are as follows:

- Personal history of depression
- Previous family history of depression
- Pressures about being a parent
- Feeling overwhelmed with expectations and your role as a father
- Financial problems
- Lack of support from society or family
- Stress in relationships with their family
- Stressful birthing experience
- Lack of sleep due to baby
- Feeling excluded from the mother-baby bond
- Lack of a good male role model
- Low testosterone

## Do fathers undergo any changes before their child is born?

Fathers also change during the period of pregnancy. This is a phenomenon that also occurs in mice. After mating, males have an increased level of vasopressin that is caused by an increase in their protective behavior. Vasopressin mediates their behavior so well that they take care of their partners by fighting off intruders.

In humans, vasopressin also plays a role. In studies where the father was given vasopressin through a nasal spray, their neural activity changed after hearing the sound of a baby crying. This suggests that vasopressin also plays a part in responding to those situations where fathers take action to protect their children.

## Effects of Postpartum Depression in Fathers

A father's mood has a big impact on his baby and partner. If a father is depressed, then they are more likely to hit their children or partner. They cannot develop a positive environment with their children where they can play games with them or sings songs as normal fathers do.

Children who grow up with aggressive fathers often face many problems in their future because of a traumatic childhood. Research has shown that a father's depression early in their child's life often puts the child in a situation where the child suffers from developmental delays.

If the father is depressed then it will also affect their relationship with their partner, which will then cause depression in their partner too.

# Video Feedback Interventions

Video feedback is a very activity in which parents' interaction with their children are recorded in video format, whether they are playing or reading a book together. Then parents sit with their therapist and the video together. They are then asked to notice their baby's behavior while they are playing with them. This makes parents more sensitive to their child and helps to establish a stronger bond.

Ultrasounds are also a great way to start to forge the father-baby bond from prenatally. During the scanning, fathers are invited to massage the abdomen of their wives and are asked to sing a song for their baby out loud.

It's amazing how babies respond to it. When the father is singing o reading a book, babies turn their heads towards the sound in the mother's womb and parents can feel the movement by touching the abdomen.

Most of us think that a baby only comes alive when it's out of the womb but we tend to forget that it is a living human being that is inside the womb long before it comes out.

Video interventions in future

We have to strive to find ways through which we can support parents even more in the future. It is now clear that prenatal and postnatal changes do play a part in changing the behavior that is mediated by hormonal and neural changes. And these interventions can be done on a big scale without being costly and can help many parents.

This could be very helpful to parents who need help improve their parenting skills. Now fathers show more support in parenting and with the help of video feedback (ultrasound), they with be able to develop their relationship with the baby even before the birth.

## Postpartum Can Occur Even in Adoptive Parents

People often talk about "baby blues" but the emotions of adoptive parents are never taken into consideration. The majority of adoptive parents also suffer from postpartum when the baby is taken to their home. They experience a big change in their life and family circle which causes anxiety in them. Many adoptive parents have shared that they do not feel the same support and do not feel the same pleasure as birth parents do. The signs and symptoms are the same as parents who have given birth to their children—experiences such as depression, loss of appetite, loss of pleasure in activities, decreased sleep and so on.

Post-adoption affects the child in the same way as it affects parents. Adoptive parents can display feelings of inadequacy, and will suffer from severe depression if they don't feel that their bond with their child is growing.

# Screening for Father's Postpartum

As it is recommended by AAP that mothers should have full routine screening during their pregnancy, fathers should also start screening using the EPDS questionnaire. Early identification of depressed fathers has helped them to remain in their present and has supported them so that they can get involved with their families.

Research has shown that it is very important for postpartum fathers to get treated as soon as possible. For becoming a good father it's important to first take care of yourself. It is very clear that PPD has many adverse consequences but there is no doubt that it is still treatable. Recognizing that the father is suffering from PPD and getting treatment can improve the quality of life for both father and mother and can decrease the risk of many problems in their children whether they are emotional or behavioral. There are a number of ways to treat PPD in fathers, including:

- Talk therapy
- Antidepressants
- Treat it like its New Year's Day
- Finding other people with PPD
- Adjust priorities

Talk therapy

Talk therapy helps postpartum fathers too. This is because sometimes just talking about something or crying it out can prove to be the best medicine. For this purpose, you don't necessarily have to talk just to your therapist but your family or friends as well. The idea is to find people you can trust and that you are sure will understand your situation.

Antidepressants

If talk therapy does not work the doctors will resort to medication. Talk with your doctor about your symptoms so they can prescribe the best antidepressants for you.

Treat it like its New Year's Day

Remember how you make New Year's resolution before the start of a new year? You always want to start a new year with more energy and a better perspective. Similarly, when a new baby is born you should also make a fresh start in your life.

Finding other people with PPD

Postpartumen.com is known to be a very popular site for information on PPD. In this site, there are many articles to which you can relate and can get information regarding your problem with its possible solution. There is also a forum available through which you can interact with other people who are going through the same situation and you can share your experience with them.

It is normal to be nervous about becoming a dad. You always want do your best to become a good father. If you are dealing with PPD then it does not make you a bad father. This situation is not your fault. But the best way to deal with it is to get proper treatment without delay.

### Adjust priorities

Mothers aren't the only ones who need to adjust their priorities after the birth of a new baby but fathers as well. In fact, it is a golden chance for a father to show his affection for both mother and baby. In an idea scenario, the father would get maternity leave from work, but if he doesn't, then he should adjust his schedule so that he can spend more time with his family and get attached to the baby. If both partners raise their child as a team, then they will be surprised to see the confidence in their children when they become adults and, in this way, they can both overcome postpartum depression together.

# Chapter 6: Problems Faced in Postpartum and Their Solutions

## Problems in Postpartum

Becoming a mother is a huge new chapter in a woman's life, and only mothers experience the joy and excitement of giving birth to a baby. Some women may struggle with mental health problems during the period of their pregnancy and after giving birth to their child. The transition of a woman into motherhood may lead to different mental health disorders such as anxiety, depression or obsessive-compulsive disorder. In addition to this, many women also face severe mental health conditions called postpartum psychosis which mostly appear after giving birth to a child. Women experience different types of feelings during the time of their pregnancy and even after giving birth to their child. After becoming the mother, all women face emotional and physical changes that can impact them differently. It is very important to identify certain changes after becoming a mother or it will lead to severe psychological problems. Postpartum depressions in new mothers is normal and there is nothing to blame yourself for. Such feelings of excitement, joy, anxiety, or depression are normal and occur naturally to every new mother. Changes in women after giving birth to a baby can be separated into two major categories which are emotional changes and physical changes.

# Emotional changes

The feelings and emotions of every human being are directly linked with mental health. People interpret different situations and conditions according to their state of mind. When a person enters into a new relationship or experiences any life change, their mental state and way of thinking also change. They are natural and normal but one has to differentiate between negative and positive thoughts. Negative thoughts can lead to anxiety and depression while positive thoughts are good for mental health. During or after the pregnancy, women undergo certain psychological phases that have a different impact on their mental wellbeing.

<u>Mood swings</u>

Mood swings and change in behavior is normal for many mothers. Mothers can't be happy and excited all the time. Entering into the world of motherhood requires few changes to their existing lifestyle. It is not easy to make changes these changes and as result women mostly feel uncomfortable in the first few weeks of motherhood. Some women also find difficult to express their feelings after giving birth to their child. New mothers mostly find it difficult to keep a stable mood, too. For example, they suddenly become sad or depressed while playing with their babies. So, if you note that you're experiencing mood swings, try to remain calm. This will help you in understanding your mental state. To overcome this situation, you can either divert your attention or consult with a specialist.

Difficulty sleeping

Sleeping patterns of many new mothers are disturbed after giving birth to the child. It is very rare that a baby will sleeps through the night or accommodate you while you're sleeping. Babies mostly sleep and wake up according to their own timings. You cannot adjust your sleep or routine according to your baby's timings, so, many mothers find it hard to complete their sleeping hours which makes them tired throughout the day. Lack of sleep also affects the mental and physical health of the mothers. To maintain your health, it is important that you should complete your sleep.

The best way to complete your sleep is during those times when your baby is also sleeping. If you have a partner, you can also get help from them by asking them to take care of the baby while you are resting.

Irritability

Nursing a newborn baby is a fulltime job that requires complete dedication. You have to fully commit yourself to your baby so that they can get all the nourishment and attention. This is a lot of work and it severely affects the mother's personal space and life. Many women become so occupied that they literally find no time for themselves. This creates discomfort and irritability for new mothers and they start disliking motherhood. Before you become irritated by your baby, you should seek help. In this regard, your partner can accommodate you. Ask your partner to spare some time from their routine and take responsibility for the baby. This will give you free time and space to relax. So, don't get exhausted by taking all the burden of your child.

Accepting a new relationship

After getting the news of being pregnant, women start accepting the new relationship of being a mother. Carrying the baby for nine months can give you feelings of care and love. After giving birth to your child, there are chances that you may feel distressed and occupied all the time. This is the time when you have to think differently and dedicate yourself to motherhood. If you are facing problems in nourishing your child then never hesitate to seek professional help. To give the best attention and care, you can take nursing or baby care classes. Being a mother is a full-time job which can be done successfully if you are well prepared. Discussing your problems with other mothers can also help you a lot in finding the best solution. So, prepare yourself completely during the months of pregnancy and welcome your newborn with an open heart.

Anxiety

For some women, giving birth to a baby is the most amazing experience of their lives. Welcoming a baby into this world brings joy and excitement in a parent's life as it completes them by making a family. Some mothers may feel down or up or want to weep after giving birth to the child. Such feelings are natural and common among women and usually last for a few weeks after the birth of the baby. These feelings are known as "baby blues". These symptoms or feelings become alarming when they prolong for longer periods and start interfering in the process of your baby care. This is the time when you should become alert as it can be postpartum depression which can lead to anxiety disorder.

Identifying the problem of depression and anxiety in the initial stage is crucial for its effective treatment. Never feel guilty or embarrassed to express your feelings. Many women face such kind of problems after giving birth to the child. Seek professional help and start treating your problem of anxiety before it gets worse.

Obsessive-compulsive disorder

Obsessive-compulsive disorder during the stages of pregnancy and after giving birth to the child is mostly ignored and misunderstood by many parents. Perinatal anxiety is common and natural among many parents after having a baby. A lot of people not diagnosed with OCD still face the symptoms of anxiety disorder. According to a study, it is estimated that about 3-5 % of new parents experience the symptoms of obsessive-compulsive disorder. These frightening and repetitive feelings of anxiety and depression can cause psychological problems. In such a phase, parents constantly experience negative thoughts and spend their time in a delusional world where they feel that anything can harm their newborn child.

Major symptoms of the postpartum obsessive-compulsive disorder include obsessions, compulsions, feelings of fear, and being overprotective for the infant. In the state of obsession, the person gets constant and repetitive negative thoughts and images of their new baby. Such feelings upset the parents and they start getting worried and stressed. Compulsion is a state in which the parent performs certain tasks again and again to overcome their obsessions and fear. Such activities mainly include counting and reordering things, cleaning constantly, or checking things many times. These symptoms are normal in the first few weeks but if this condition prolongs to months then it needs professionals for treatment.

## Lack of concentration

After the birth of a child, most mothers spend their time nourishing their newborns. It is natural and normal to give full attention and care to the baby. Many women take leave from their professional responsibilities so that they can take care of their newborn. In the first few weeks of childbirth, it is not possible to divert your attention and care from your child.

## Lost interest in sex

During the period of pregnancy, women undergo a unique mental state. New mothers mostly experience different feelings like fear, stress, joy, excitement and sadness at the same time. Refraining from sex during the months of pregnancy reduces interest in sex. So, after giving birth to the baby most women show less or no interest in sex. Don't blame yourself, it is common and natural. To overcome such feelings, spend some alone time with your partner without having your baby around.

### Intrusive thoughts

Unpleasant and unwelcoming thoughts are known as intrusive thoughts. These thoughts are the basic reason for stress and can cause panic attacks. During the period of pregnancy and postpartum, most women spend a lot of time alone with their babies. In these moments, their mind's may become flooded with intrusive thoughts.


### Confusion

Only a healthy and active mind is able to make correct decisions. After giving birth to a child almost every woman undergoes certain psychological problems which can cause anxiety and depression. Random thoughts and anxiety hinder their thought process. This is why most women in labor seem confused. They mostly take some time in giving an answer to a simple question. This phase of confusion lasts for a few days and you will start feeling normal after this period.


### Hallucination

The most severe psychological problem after childbirth is hallucinations. Their partner should closely observe the condition of the new mother and if hallucinations are taking place, then immediately consult a psychiatrist. Normally such a severe condition doesn't prolong for more than a few days.

Disorganized behavior

Family members and friends start feeling worried when they see sudden behavioral changes in new mothers. New start feeling irritated about small things, preoccupied, over-possessive of the baby. These negative thoughts affect the behavior of new mothers and they start behaving strangely. These minor behavioral changes are normal and new mothers overcome such emotions with the passage of time. These psychological problems don't need any medication or treatment. Entering into the new world of motherhood is an entirely different experience for most women.

## Physical Changes

Besides emotional changes, women do face certain prominent physical changes after giving birth to the child. These charges vary from person to person and according to the type of their body. Some changes are temporary while some will be permanent. Nourishing another being's life in your womb for nine months requires you to be physically healthy. Your body will sacrifice its energy, nutrients and other important minerals while you are pregnant. This means that you have to take extra care of yourself during the months of pregnancy.

The process of delivery may be easy or complicated. You can either have a vaginal delivery or cesarean birth (C-section) depending upon the condition of your pregnancy. It doesn't matter which type of delivery you have gone through, your body has still given birth to a baby which means that you may have to stay in labor for a few hours or for few days. The recovery phase may take some time. It will take some time to completely recover from the process of postpartum. Normally, it takes a few months to fully recover from pregnancy and childbirth. The average period for recovery is 6-8 weeks but it may take longer in some cases. During the recovery phase, you will find your body unresponsive or unsupportive. Try to remain calm and don't get frustrated. This is the time to get maximum rest, eat well and healthy and give your body a break. Keep in mind that your body is not aware of your expectations and will become normal after completing the recovery phase.

After giving birth to a child, your body may experience following physical changes.

Abdominal pain

You will experience abdomen (lower belly) pain when your uterus shrinks back into normal shape and size after giving birth to a baby. Such pains are known as "after pains". The intensity of these pains is mostly dull and low but they can also be sharp sometimes. During the time of breastfeeding, such pains may occur frequently and with high intensity. This happens because while breastfeeding, your body will produce a chemical that affects the uterus and helps it to contract. To control the intensity of the pain, you can use a heating pad or warm water bottle in the painful area. This will help in reducing your abdominal pain. If the pain continues and gets worse, consult with your doctor.

Hair problems

One of the positive side-effects of pregnancy is denser and lusher hair. During the period of pregnancy, women experience hair growth and find their hair thicker. This is due to hormonal changes in the body. After the birth of a child, hormones levels start returning to normal which will cause the luscious hair to fall off. Don't panic, you will not become bald. You will experience the problem of hair loss in the early months of postpartum which will eventually stop and your hair will become normal again. Avoid using harmful haircare and skincare products during the months of pregnancy and nursing as it can pass into the bloodstream and then into your growing baby. Always use organic hair care and skincare products especially when you are pregnant and nursing your baby.

Changes in breasts size

You will observe a clear difference in your breast size after giving birth to your child. The bras which you have purchased during the period of your pregnancy will no longer fit you. This is because estrogen and progesterone levels drop after the childbirth and another hormone, prolactin, kicks in that helps in producing breast milk. This hormonal change produces extra milk in your breasts which makes them bigger. This happens because of increased blood and milk flow. After two to three days from delivery, you will feel your breasts sore and hard. This problem will be resolved naturally if you're breastfeeding your baby. You can also use additional methods to reduce the hardness of your breasts, which include applying warm packs to your breasts before feeding and cold packs afterward. You can take mild anti-inflammatory medication such as ibuprofen which is safe during breastfeeding.

In case you are not breastfeeding your baby, then the breast engorgement may take a week or two to resolve. In the meantime, you can use a snug bra, ice packs and ibuprofen to get ease the discomfort and pain.

## Vitamins and minerals

You may feel exhausted and shaky in the first few weeks after the delivery. Multiple wake-ups in the middle of the night, feelings of low energy and feeling reluctant to perform normal tasks are the common symptoms of iron deficiency. There is a high risk of low iron levels in the new moms which are mostly caused due to blood loss during the process of delivering the child. This is a very common problem in many new mothers and can be controlled by following a dietitian's advice. Iron deficiency can be resolved by taking prenatal multivitamins with iron, especially when you are breastfeeding. Even if you are not breastfeeding, it is still recommended that you take multivitamins with iron. In addition to this, you should also eat iron-rich foods such as beans, red meat, fortified whole-grain products, leafy greens and lentils. Once your iron levels start rising, you will start feeling normal and energetic. Some severe deficiencies such as shortness of breath, dizziness, pale skin, a swollen tongue, cold and/or hot hands and feet may take longer to resolve. To check iron levels in your body, your doctor will ask you for some blood tests.

The vitamins that your body requires while you are breastfeeding include vitamin A, C, E, and B complex with copper, chlorine, chromium, iodine, zinc, and selenium. The best and easiest way to overcome any deficiencies of the above vitamins and minerals is through a healthy diet. Eat healthy foods that contain high protein levels and complex carbohydrates such as fruits, certain veggies and whole grain. Some researchers also claim that vitamin D deficiency is a major cause of postpartum mood disorders. Always ask your doctor first before taking any supplements.

Stitches

In case you had to get stitches due to a cut or torn perineum, it will take 7-10 days to heal. Depending on the material used for the stitches, you will observe that they will disappear over time. To keep the stitches safe from infection gently wash the area with warm water after using the toilet each time. A squirt bottle can be used to rinse the area and dry it gently. Try to keep your hands away from the stitches no matter how desperate you are to check the healing progress. In case you are feeling pain in the stitches or they seem to be leaking, contact your doctor immediately. Leaking and painful stitches could be a sign of infection.

The stitches of a C-section vary in healing. It takes 5-10 days to heal stitches which are on the surface of your skin. It will take longer to heal stitches that are underneath your skin, in your muscles for example. Muscles stitches can take more than 12 weeks to completely heal. Visible stitches should be observed carefully to make sure that they are safe from infection. Common indications of infection include redness, pus, swollen skin or in some cases you may feel fever.

# Chapter 7: Vaginal Discharge

It is common to face the problem of vaginal discharge (also known as lochia) and bleeding after giving birth to your child. This is not a problem to worry about as all this blood and tissue was used to grow and nourish your baby. After childbirth, your body eliminates all the extra blood and other material out from your body. In the first 10 days after childbirth, you can expect to have heavier vaginal bleeding and discharge but it will gradually decrease. You can expect light bleeding and discharge up to six weeks after the delivery. It is recommended to use only sanitary pads during this period. The application of tampons can cause bacteria and infection. Some clots can also be expected in the first week. If the clots keep on coming and become bigger in size, you should consult with your doctor immediately.

## Weight problems

After giving birth to your baby, your weight will probably go down. You are expected to lose between 4-6 pounds of pure water weight during the first week after birth alone. This is mainly caused due to increased sweating and urination. Breastfeeding mothers are expected to lose even more weight. 300-500 extra calories burned a day as a result of nursing a bay. Breastfeeding will make you feel hungrier and can also be the reason for weight loss.

## Constipation

Postpartum constipation can be caused due to various reasons such as dehydration, having a C-section, side-effects of pain medication and fear of pushing something out of your body after delivery. New mothers are prone to face postpartum constipation in the first week. You can handle the problem of postpartum constipation by drinking lots of water, drinking In the worst-case scenario, your doctor or nurse may also prescribe you a stool softener to overcome the problem of constipation.

## Pelvic floor and bladder problems

In case you pee a little in your pants while laughing, sneezing or exercise then it is a clear indication that your pelvic floor needs some care and attention. This condition is normal in many new mothers after the childbirth and continues for a few days or weeks. The pelvic floor includes the tissues, muscles, ligaments and nerves that provide support to your vagina, bladder, uterus and rectum. The pelvic floor undergoes a lot of stress and pressure during the process of delivery, labor and the weight of the baby. You can treat this problem with the help of pelvic health physiotherapy. The pelvic floor becomes weak after the child's delivery or after facing any injury.

A most common issue which can be faced after pregnancy is bladder incontinence and occasionally you can also face the problem of fecal incontinence (leaking poo). Prolapse can also be caused as a result of a damaged pelvic floor. This weakens the vaginal wall which can cause rectum, bladder or uterus to drop from the original position.

You can identify this situation by analyzing its symptoms such as pain during sex, frequent peeing or pee leaks or a feeling of pressure in your lower abdomen.

The best way to strengthen the pelvic floor is through physiotherapy. It can teach you how to perform certain exercises to build up the pelvic muscles. Pelvic floor assessment is usually done after six weeks after delivery.

After childbirth, core abdomen muscles become weakened which makes it difficult to lift things after pregnancy. Almost all new mothers will face the problem of diastasis recti, which is a gap between the left abdominal wall muscles and the right abdomen wall muscles. The reason behind this problem is again hormones that weaken the muscle tissue. Usually, in the first eight weeks after childbirth, this gap between the muscles is filled up automatically. In case the gap remains, then you will still look like you're pregnant, can face back pain problems and will face difficulty in pushing, pulling and lifting things. In this kind of situation, a pelvic physiotherapist can guide you and teach you the right exercises that can help in regaining the strength of the abdominal muscles. Keeping the problem of diastasis recti aside, many women end up with a floppier and softer tummy after childbirth. This mainly depends upon the genetics, types of skin tissues and how you carry yourself.

# Pain in the perineal area

Mothers can deliver a child in two ways. One is vaginal delivery and the second one is cesarean delivery. The perineal area is the specific area from where the baby comes out of the mother's womb. It is quite a painful process to push a 7-8 pounds—or sometimes bigger—baby through a small opening. So, it is natural and common to feel some pain and tenderness in your perineal area after child delivery. The amount of perineal pain and its recovery is entirely dependent upon the method of delivery and also on the person. Some common things which you can expect from your perineal area:

Vaginal tear or an episiotomy: It will take approximately 7-10 days to heal the wound. For the next 6 weeks or maybe more, it will feel sensitive and sore.

Vaginal birth: After giving birth to the child, the rectum and the entire perineal area will be swollen. For around three to five weeks, you will feel discomfort in this area.

By adopting some precautionary measures, you can reduce irritation and discomfort in your perineal area.

Try to keep your perineal area clean: After urinating, use warm water with a squirt bottle over the torn skin. This will reduce the irritation and keep your sensitive area clean and safe from infection.

Use ice packs: For soothing relief and to reduce the swelling, use a crushed ice compress or a maxi pad equipped with a cold pack.

Apply the cold to the site by putting an interval of a few hours during the first 48 hours.

Heat the painful area: Sitting in a tub containing warm water will also reduce the discomfort and irritation. Dip your hips and buttocks in warm water for at least 20 minutes. Perform this activity a few times a day to get ease from pain and discomfort.

Numb the area: In case of severe pain, you can also use local anesthetics in the form of creams, sprays, pads or ointments as prescribed by your doctor. This will give you immediate relief from pain. Acetaminophen (Tylenol) can also be used.

Ease the pressure: Try to divert the pressure from your sore perineum by changing your posture. Avoid sitting or standing for long periods and try to sleep and lie on your side whenever possible. Use an inflated tube (usually prescribed to hemorrhoid sufferers) or a pillow (with an opening in the center) for sitting. It will help in strengthening and tightening your buttock muscles.

Use loose clothes: Use loose and free size clothing (like sweat pants, baggy trousers) to let your perineum breathe. Tight-fitting clothes and underwear can cause irritation., which will slow down the process of healing.

## Change in body size

During the phase of pregnancy, it is not just your abdomen that increases in size, but other parts of your body also. Your baby develops in your body during the nine months of pregnancy, which causes your ribcage and uterus to expand. To provide easy access to the birth canal, you will also notice that your hips become widened. After giving birth to your child, you may feel that your hips and ribcage may not go back to the same shape as they used to be before the pregnancy. According to some new mothers, it is really hard to get the same shape back even after returning to the same pre-baby weight.

## **A Short message from Mommy's Angels:**

Hey, are you enjoying the book? I'd love to hear your thoughts! Many readers do not know how hard reviews are to come by, and how much they help an author.

I would be incredibly thankful if you could take just 60 seconds to write a brief review on Amazon, even if it's just a few sentences!

\>> Click here to leave a quick review

Thank you for taking the time to share your thoughts!

Your review will genuinely make a difference for me and help gain exposure for my work.

# Chapter 8: Preventive Measures for Postpartum

It is natural to face certain emotional and physical problems after giving birth to your child. New mothers mostly become confused and stressed after facing unexpected problems during the period of postpartum. You can overcome such problems by following these simple steps.

## Meditation

Mental wellbeing plays a crucial role in the physical health of a person. Being a new mother is an entirely new chapter in a woman's life. It can cause stress and anxiety in a woman's mind that can make her physically weak. At the same time, mothers also experience a feeling of excitement and joy. During the phase of postpartum, it is very important to feel relaxed and enjoy all the moments with your newborn baby. New mothers can control their feelings and mind through meditation. Meditation plays an important role in the development of the human mind and teaches a person how to enter into a deep state of relaxation. Meditation reduces fatigue and stress, overcome generalized anxiety disorder, and treat people who are suffering from insomnia and other psychological problems.

New mothers should learn the techniques of meditation to overcome their mental state of anxiety and depression. Some popular techniques of meditation include mindfulness meditation, loving-kindness meditation, body-scan or progressive relaxation, Zen meditation, Transcendental meditation, Kundalini yoga, and Breath awareness meditation. You should choose one technique of meditation that suits you best and start treating your problem of anxiety.

## Placenta Therapy

During pregnancy, a special organ is developed in the uterus known as the placenta. The basic purpose of this organ is to provide nutrients and oxygen to your developing baby and remove waste from the baby's blood. One end of placenta attaches to your baby's umbilical cord and the other end to the wall of the uterus. The placenta attaches to the front, back, side or top of the uterus. In some cases, you will also find this organ attached to the lower uterine region that is known as placenta previa. Possible placenta complications during pregnancy may include placenta previa, placenta accreta and placental abruption. Heavy vaginal bleeding can be caused because of these problems. Retained placenta after childbirth may also cause some problems such as:

**Retained Placenta**: Retained placenta is the amount of placenta that is not delivered within 30 minutes after childbirth. The reason behind placenta retention is that the placenta may be trapped behind the partially closed cervix due to its attachment to the uterine wall either deeply or loosely. Left untreated, retained placenta can cause life-threatening blood loss or severe infection.

**Placenta Accreta**: This is a serious condition related to placenta complication. Placenta accreta is a condition where the blood vessels and related parts of the placenta grow deeply into the uterine wall. Normally, the placenta is automatically removed from the uterine wall after the childbirth but in placenta accreta, the parts remain attached to the uterine wall. This particular condition can cause severe blood loss after childbirth. In such a scenario, your doctor may recommend the removal of your uterus (hysterectomy) to save your life. In rare cases, the placenta penetrates into the uterus muscles (placenta increta) or grows the uterine wall (placenta percreta).

**Placenta Previa**: Placenta previa is a condition when the cervix (the outlet of uterus) is partially or totally covered by the placenta. This condition occurs in the early stages of pregnancy and can be resolved as the uterus grows. During pregnancy and child delivery, severe vaginal bleeding can be caused due to placenta previa. The treatment procedure depends on the amount of vaginal bleeding, how far along your pregnancy is, whether the bleeding stops, the exact position of the placenta and your baby's health. Your doctor may recommend a C-section if the placenta previa persists in the later stages of your pregnancy.

**Placental Abruption**: Placental abruption is a condition where the placenta is partially or completely detached from the uterus before delivery. This can interrupt the supply of oxygen and nutrients to the baby and can also cause you to bleed heavily. Early child delivery is mostly recommended by doctors when facing such a condition.

Major symptoms of placental complications mainly include abdominal pain, vaginal bleeding, uterine contractions and back pain. There are no direct treatment options to overcome placental problems, but by following few precautionary measures, you can avoid complications.

- Regularly visit your doctor to get thoroughly checked during the period of your pregnancy
- Inform your doctor immediately if you are facing any unexpected problems like high blood pressure
- Avoid smoking and taking any illegal or unprescribed drugs during your pregnancy
- Consult with your doctor before deciding on a C-section delivery
- If you faced a placental problem in a previous pregnancy and are planning to get pregnant again, inform your doctor before your pregnancy. Take regular advice from your doctor to avoid any placenta complications in your next pregnancy.

## Acupuncture and acupressure

Acupuncture and acupressure are ancient Chinese techniques that are used to treat people who are suffering from emotional, mental and physical problems. In acupuncture, small needles are used to puncture the skin in specific spots to overcome illness and physiological issues. Modern medical science also believes in this method of treatment because needles are inserted into the specific nerves which help in increasing the blood flow and nerve stimulation process.

During pregnancy, many women face morning tiredness or sickness and feel unable to move. To overcome this condition, pregnant women mostly purchase sea bands that are in the form of wrist bracelets. These bands provide relief and reduce the effects of morning sickness or motion sickness by targeting specific pressure points of the wrist. Most women also consider applying acupressure techniques during their initial days of labor. These techniques are also used to help induce labor on its own, without applying external methods. The best way to apply acupressure is through foot massages at or near the due date. The pleasant pain of a foot massage will divert your attention from your contraction and help you to get relaxed.

After giving birth to the baby, acupressure can help you in alleviating various problems like postpartum depression, back pain, lactation, hip pain, mastitis, sciatica, tiredness, exhaustion, and urinary incontinence. The process of growing and delivering a baby consumes a huge amount of the mother's energy and nutrients. During pregnancy and labor, your body will produce a hormone known as relaxin, which loosens up the body muscles especially hips to provide you support. Many women also complain about sciatica, which is caused due to the weight of the baby on the sciatic nerve. You can overcome all these postpartum issues through applying the techniques of acupressure. These techniques will help you in getting relief from almost all kinds of postpartum pains.

**Motherwort**

Motherwort (Leonurus cardiaca) was used by the ancient Greeks to overcome the feelings of anxiety after childbirth. Due to its potential properties, motherwort is primarily used as a tincture or tea.

Motherwort looks like a straight upright stem with a prickly bush of dark green leaves and fuzzy purple or pink flowers on top. Initially, this plant was only found in Asia and Southeastern Europe, but is now available worldwide. It belongs to the family of mint herbs but has a bitter flavor and unpleasant smell. Motherwort is considered to be effective against anxiety, heart disease and irregular menstruation.

Various other health benefits can also be attained by using herbs. Numerous plant-based antioxidant compounds can be found in motherwort, such as sterols, flavonoids, triterpenes, and tannins. These antioxidants compounds can protect your cells from harmful chemicals known as free radicals. Studies have shown that antioxidants can also keep you safe from several deadly problems such as heart disease, Parkinson's, cancer, Alzheimer's and arthritis.

Potential benefits of Motherwort may include blood loss recovery during child delivery, alleviating the anxiety during the period of postpartum, and may also decrease inflammation. Motherwort is a natural herb which means that there is no restriction in its usage. To avoid any possible side-effects, you can also consult with your doctor before starting.

## Prenatal Vitamins

Prenatal vitamins contain almost all kinds of important minerals and vitamins that are considered necessary for new mothers. These minerals and vitamins mainly include Calcium, Iron, Folic Acid, and Iodine. All these minerals and vitamins will fulfill your body requirements and will provide a healthy environment for your baby to develop and grow. The bones of the mother and baby will get stronger with the help of Calcium. Iron will help in carrying oxygen through the blood of both mom and baby. You can start taking prenatal vitamins even before conception. During the initial months of pregnancy, these vitamins will play a vital role in the development of your baby. The baby's brain and spinal cord (also known as a neural tube) develop during the first month of your pregnancy. So, it is beneficial for you to increase the intake of folic acid which will ease the baby's development.

**Avoid Being Alone**

The worst thing you can encounter during your pregnancy and even after giving birth is boredom. Spending time alone can stagnate your mind and you will start feeling depressed. This can even lead to anxiety disorder. New mothers mostly have an ample amount of free time, which is normally hard to pass. This problem can be tackled by managing your activities. Manage your time in such a way that you will have no free time to sit alone and idle. Try to spend as much time as you can with your newborn baby. It will keep you involved with your baby. You can also ask your partner to spend more time with you and try to communicate as much as you can with them. Chatting with a friend on a phone can also help in passing your idle time. So, whenever you find yourself alone and free immediately engage yourself in any activity that you enjoy.

## Maintain Your Diet

It is important to provide complete nourishment to the developing baby. Pregnant women should maintain a balanced diet to get maximum energy. Foods that are considered to be beneficial during the months of pregnancy are sweet potatoes, legumes, dairy products, eggs, salmon, broccoli, fish liver oil, berries, whole grains, avocados, dried fruit, water, and lean meat. During pregnancy, you may need to take 350-500 calories extra on a daily basis to fulfill the requirements of your body and baby. Weight gain and poor diet plans can make complications in childbirth and can also increase the risk of gestational diabetes.

Dairy Products: Extra calcium and proteins are required during the months of pregnancy. Dairy products can help you in getting two types of high-quality protein: whey and casein. Other important components which can be attained through dairy products are Calcium, Zinc, Phosphorus, Magnesium, and Vitamin B. For pregnant women, yogurt is quite beneficial. It supports digestive health as it contains probiotic bacteria. Probiotic supplements can greatly reduce the risk of childbirth complications such as gestational diabetes, preeclampsia, vaginal infection and allergies.

Sweet Potatoes: Beta-carotene is found in sweet potatoes, which is a plant compound that turns into vitamin A when enters the human body. Vitamin A plays an important role in the growth of various body cells and tissues. It also contributes to fetal development. Pregnant women should take 10-40% more vitamin A than women who are not pregnant. High amounts of an animal-based sources of vitamin A should be avoided, as it is highly toxic and it can be harmful to the baby. The best source of getting vitamin A is through beta-carotene. Pregnant women should take about 3.5-5.3 ounces of cooked sweet potatoes to fulfill their daily requirements. Sweet potatoes can also provide you with fiber which can help in digestion and reduce blood sugar levels.

Legumes: Peas, lentils, beans, soybeans, chickpeas, and peanuts are a good source of plant-based protein, fiber, calcium, iron and folate (B9). These are the primary requirements of your body during the months of pregnancy. Folate belongs to the family of B vitamins (B9) which is crucial for the health of the fetus and mother. Insufficient folate intake can lead to various complications such as low birth weight and increased risk of neural tube defects. High amounts of folate can be obtained from legumes. It is estimated that one cup of black beans, lentils or chickpeas can provide 65-90% of the folate needed. A high amount of fiber, magnesium, iron and zinc can also be obtained from legumes.

Eggs: Eggs take the top position in the list of healthy food items. It contains almost every nutrient required by the body on a daily basis. Eggs contain high-quality fat, protein, calories, minerals and vitamins. Your body can also get choline from eggs, which is beneficial in the development of your body including the brain. During pregnancy, low choline intake can cause the risk of neural tube defects which can affect the brain functioning in the fetus. A large egg contains approximately 113 mg of choline.

Salmon: You can get essential omega-3 fatty acids from salmon. Most pregnant women fail to get enough omega-3 through their daily diet. Omega-3 fatty acids are important especially during pregnancy. High amounts of omega-3 acids can be found in seafood. These acids help in developing the brain and eyes of your fetus. Pregnant women should limit seafood to twice a week in order to avoid mercury poisoning and other contaminants in fatty fish. Studies suggest that to fulfill the requirements of omega-3 fatty acids, pregnant women should eat 2-3 meals of fatty fish per week. To get vitamin D naturally, salmon is the only way. Vitamin D is required by many processes of your body like immune function and bone health. Most of your daily diet plan lacks in providing you required vitamin D.

Lean meat: Pure, high-quality protein can be obtained from fish, chicken, and beef. Beef is a rich source of choline, iron and other B vitamins which are highly needed during the period of pregnancy. Iron is a crucial mineral used by red blood cells to maintain hemoglobin. It also plays an important role in providing oxygen to all cells within your body. Pregnant women require more iron due to increased blood volume. Insufficient levels of iron in the woman's body may cause pregnancy complications such as the risk of premature delivery, iron deficiency anemia and low birth weight. With the help of diet alone it may become hard for a pregnant woman to overcome the iron deficiency of the body. This is because most pregnant women start disliking meat during their pregnancy. Women who regularly eat red meat may obtain the required levels of iron from their diet. Vitamin C enriched foods play an important role in increasing the absorption of iron from meals. Oranges or bell peppers are the rich sources of getting vitamin C.

Fish liver oil: Fish liver oil is rich in omega-3 fatty acids and vitamin D. Lack of vitamin D increases the risk of preeclampsia, a complicated problem that can be diagnosed through identifying its symptoms such as swelling of the hands and feet, high blood pressure and protein in the urine. During the early stages of pregnancy, you should consume cod liver oil to help the baby in gaining weight and also to decrease the risk of disease in a baby's life. One tablespoon (approximately 15 ml) of fish liver oil can fulfill your daily need of vitamin A, vitamin D and omega-3. It is not recommended to consume more than one tablespoon of fish liver oil. High levels of preformed vitamin A in your body can be dangerous for your fetus. Increased levels of omega-3 can have blood-thinning effects.

Berries: Berries are rich in healthy carbs, vitamin C, water, fiber, and antioxidants. Appropriate levels of vitamin C helps the body to absorb iron. It is also important for skin health and helps the immune system to work efficiently. Berries will not increase your blood sugar levels as they have a low glycemic index value. Berries can provide you with fiber and water, which makes them a healthy snack. With a relatively low level of calories, berries can provide a good flavor and nutrition.

Avocados: They contain high levels of monounsaturated fatty acids, vitamin K, D vitamins (especially folate), fiber, potassium, copper, vitamin E, and vitamin C. High amounts of healthy fats like potassium and folate make avocados beneficial for pregnant women. The healthy fats of avocados help in developing the brain, tissues and skin of your fetus and folate protect the neural tube from defects. Potassium-filled avocados help in getting relief from leg cramps which are a normal side effect of pregnancy for some women. Avocados contain even more potassium than bananas.

Whole grains: Requirement of calories and other major nutrients are increased in pregnant women especially during the second and third month. Whole grain food items can fulfill your body's needs. Refined grains lack almost all major components like vitamins, fiber and plant compounds which can only be obtained through whole grains. During pregnancy, you can eat oats and quinoa, which are full of protein.

Dried fruit: By eating dried fruits you can get high-quality fiber, calories, vitamins and minerals. Dried fruit contains the almost same amount of nutrients as fresh fruit but without having any water. A single serving of dried fruit is can give you a high quantity of minerals, vitamins, folate, iron and potassium. Prunes are a rich source of sorbitol, vitamin K, potassium and fiber. It can also help you in overcoming constipation. Dates can provide you with plant compounds, potassium, iron and fiber.

Water: It is very important to keep your body properly hydrated, especially during pregnancy because your blood volume increases by up to 1.5 liters. Your developing baby will get all the nutrients but you have to keep your water levels maintained or else you may become dehydrated. Mild dehydration symptoms mainly include anxiety, headache, tiredness, a bad mood and poor memory. With an appropriate level of water intake, you can prevent constipation and reduce your risk of urinary tract infections. Two liters of water is the recommended amount for a healthy body.

## Share your feelings

Postpartum depression is a phase that can be neglected or avoided by expressing your feelings. Try to be open with your family and friends and share your thoughts and feelings with them. If you have a partner, whenever you feel alone and depressed ask them to accompany you so that you can tackle your thoughts of anxiety.

**Make yourself feel special**

After having a baby, most new mothers become so busy that they never find any time for themselves. Being a mother is a full-time job that requires your complete dedication and commitment. Nourishing and taking care of your baby all the time will make you feel spent and stressed. Before this becomes a larger issue, like depression, try to spare some time for yourself. You can ask your partner or family to handle the baby for some time and in the meanwhile, you can pamper yourself.

**Exercise**

Physical exercise is the best activity to relax your body and mind. After giving birth to your child, it is very important for new mothers to start doing mild exercise. It will greatly help blood circulation, especially to the brain. During the last months of pregnancy, most women keep from doing physical activities, so it is very important to stretch your body by doing exercise.

**Stay in a positive environment**

Your surrounding environment plays an important role in the development of the human mind and personality. A person living in a positive and healthy environment will be more lively and energetic. For new mothers, it is very important to stay in a positive environment. It will help them in overcoming postpartum disorders.

# Chapter 9: Effects of Postpartum on Newborns

Postpartum depression is not only responsible for the changes in the mother's life but can also affect the growth and happiness of the newborn. Many postpartum disorders affect a new mother. Some factors that can affect the mothers are the financial issues and the confusion related to child development. The stress that a women faces will also affect her ability to care for her child and this will be problematic for the baby. You need to understand that the postpartum effects will not stop in their childhood but will stem to their entire childhood. The children who face problematic childhood will have confidence issues that can affect their personal and professional life.

## Infant Development and Mother's Depression

**Mother/newborn communication**

The mother has the closest connection with her newborn. The newborn will learn many things form the mother and if the mother/newborn relationship is not strong, this will pose a communication problem between the mother and the baby. Depression can lead to many issues between the mother and her child and the child will distance himself from the parents. This means that it will have a negative effect of its growth. The mothers who face depression are emotionally cut-off from the world and will not give proper love and care to the child. Newborns can't adapt or self-control this negative state, and create inactivity, withdrawal and self-administrative practices (e.g. turning away or sucking on thumb)

**Psychological improvement**

The psychological improvement of the babies with mothers experiencing postpartum depression is also affected. The research also displays that the babies with mothers who experience PPD have less brain development than the babies with healthy mothers. The mothers who are affected by the PPD will not offer the same love and affection to the babies. The babies get a negative vibe in the house and this affects their overall development. It has been reported that a newborn child's own negative influence meddles with learning and the capacity to process data.

# Maternal depression and developmental outcome of toddlers and preschoolers

**Conduct advancement**

The mothers who face depression after their delivery will not be able to cater to the needs of the babies. They possess a negative mindset and this critical thinking approach will affect the overall development of the child. The practices of the mothers have been studied and the effects on the children. The children who face communication issues in the start will tend to be rebellious in nature and face problems in affecting the norms of the society. They hesitate in taking part in the physical activities. These parts of kid conduct were related with postnatal gloom under unfriendly circumstances, for example, conjugal clash, and segment factors, for example, maternal age, ethnicity, financial status, conjugal status, and the child's age.

**Intellectual advancement**

The baby's intellectual development will be affected when the mother will face PPD. The mother's attention is one of the most important factor that affects the intellectual capacity of the child. Different parts of intellectual advancement, for example, subjective phonetic working have additionally been demonstrated to be contrarily influenced, and there were likewise shortfalls on the perceptual and execution scale.

# Maternal depression and developmental outcome of school-age children

The school going children who face the lack of support from the mothers will face many issues in their school life as well. The mothers who are affected by PPD will not be able to cater to the needs of the children and this will increase child aggravation. Offspring of discouraged guardians are additionally at higher danger of psychopathology, including emotional problems and stress.

Even with the impacts of constant pressure factually controlled, there are still contrasts in the psychosocial result factors in certain studies. Different studies, in which there were no segment contrasts (age, conjugal status and financial level) among discouraged and non-depressed guardians, have affirmed an expanded danger of psychopathology in the offspring of discouraged guardians. It appears that beginning of a significant despondency issue before 30 years old in guardians expands the danger of their youngsters creating melancholy during youth.

**Social advancement**

For the most part, puberty is a difficult period for mental health that is twice as frequent in teenage girls than in teenage boys. Two cross-sectional studies indicated that young people with a discouraged parent experienced psychosocial maladjustment than teenagers of nonaffective mental control guardians.

Studies have reliably detailed higher instances of significant wretchedness and other psychopathology in young people with a mentally ill, normally starting at 15 to 20 years of age.

## Role of the father figure

The role of father figures and its relationship with a developing haven't been researched as much, instead focusing on maternal figures, potentially in light of the fact that the primary guardian for the youthful newborn child is normally the mother. It has been shown however that newborn children of discouraged moms connected better with their non-depressed fathers who could ease the impacts of the postpartum disorder. What's more, a cross-sectional investigation of 96 families with kids between the ages of five and 10 years indicated that in families wherein the mother was discouraged, kids demonstrated lower social and enthusiastic capability if the dad additionally had a mental issue. The role of fathers has been considered in a roundabout way with regards to conjugal conflict, but it is known that it has a direct negative impact on a child's mental health.

## Attributes of the child

There are some distinctions in how postpartum disorders affect children based on gender. In particular, boys tend to be affected more intensely than girls.

A child's temperament likewise adds to the relational procedures of parental despondency. It has been demonstrated that depressed moms make progressively negative evaluations of their child's practices, feel less positive about their parental capabilities and utilize maladaptive child rearing methods more frequently. A child with an increasingly vigorous and accommodating disposition will be progressively impenetrable to their discouraged mother's negative conduct and won't show an equal example of cynicism. A child's strengths provide them with social and psychological aptitudes that assist them with accepting positive consideration from grown-ups other than their discouraged guardians and help lessen their discouraged parent's inclination of noncompetence and dismissal. It appears that a comprehension of the parent's sickness and acknowledgment by the child that the person in question isn't to be faulted for the parent's disease, related conduct is essential to the improvement of flexibility in a kid.

**Family treatment**

Young kids and teenagers from families with a discouraged parent may profit from family-focused therapy, concentrating on the parent's emotional problems and on the improvement of versatility in the kid. Studies have shown that the intervention of a therapist is incredibly beneficial to families suffering from these issues.

# Chapter 10: Advantage of Partner Support in Postpartum

Having a child will drastically affect the lives of the parents. There are many challenges that a woman has to face when she is facing depression after giving birth to the child. The children and the parents will have to face different mental and possibly physical challenges in their lives.

While research on postpartum disorders has focused on the sufferer of the disorder, scientists have proposed that having a partner and the elements of this relationship may be progressively significant determinants of postpartum disorders. It is believed that a safe and steady relationship assumes a significant job in adapting to the issues sooner and in a more effective way. The relationship of the couple plays a vital part in treating the PPD and in raising the child. The partner can help the woman to fight the negative thoughts in the mind and ensure that the newborn gets maximum attention. The research on the romantic couples supporting the newborn is minimal.

## Accomplice Support

The romantic connections have a strong role in one's life. These relationships are more important in hard times when a person is feeling low or they are going through depression or anxiety. The professional life can be very daunting when you have PPD. At this time, the partner support can help you cope to the pressure of the professional life. The social life is also affected when you have a supporting partner.

The period after the delivery can be eased with the help of social help. You will find many theories that support this fact. When a person has an active social circle, they will tend to find help from it when needed. During the PPD days, the social help can ease the professional pressure and the new mothers can also get help completing their chores which can be otherwise a major cause of tiredness or depression. There are many people that you can look forward in case of an emergency. You can take help from your partner, your siblings or your friends. The romantic relationships are one of the most intimate and crucial relations in one's life and this is why, having partner support during the postpartum depression is very important. The partner will feel responsible for the newborn as well and will help you to come back to your normal routine by helping your with daily chores and giving you the support you need.

The referenced qualities of the accomplice relationship recognize the accomplice support from different types of social backings that originate from various sources. There is a strong connection between the PPD and partner support. Most PPD cases were reported in women who live alone as they had no partner support. The weeks after the delivery are difficult. The women are recovering from the delivery. At this time, when a woman does not have an accomplice support, they can easily fall prey to the depression and anxiety.

Additionally, as indicated by the consequences of another examination exploring the connection between accomplice bolster evaluated a month and a half after birth and post pregnancy anxiety surveyed five months after birth, the danger of having melancholy side effects was lower in ladies with higher view of help. It is expressed that ladies who accept that they would be upheld by their accomplice and who could impart their interests to their accomplice unafraid of being scrutinized or dismissed were more averse to create manifestations of sorrow. In an investigation led in Turkey, the acquired outcomes were reliable with the past discoveries in the writing. In the referenced investigation directed with ladies who were first time moms, disappointment with fatherly help was accounted for to foresee baby blues burdensome side effects. As it were, as the fulfillment with accomplice bolster builds, the side effects of post birth anxiety decline for ladies. Predictable with the investigations indicating the impacts of apparent accomplice support on post pregnancy anxiety, the aftereffects of different examinations appear to be perfect with referenced discoveries.

The postpartum depression's signs are different in different women. Sometimes the women can show the signs after three months of delivery and this is why, the accomplice support is important. The women who face martial issues and have problems with their spouses have more chance to get PPD. Also, in another examination, disappointment with accomplice support was accounted for to be related with a more significant level of post pregnancy anxiety.

The help from society is also an important factor in helping the women with the postpartum depression. In an investigation in regards to post pregnancy anxiety, steady with the view that social help can influence melancholy in a roundabout way, it was discovered that impression of parental self-viability interceded the connection between social help and post birth anxiety. Additionally, in another investigation it was accounted for that explicitly accomplice bolster influenced peripartum melancholy (sadness during pregnancy and all through the baby blues period) both straightforwardly and by decreasing the impacts of pressure. It is viewed as that there seems a requirement for new research to more readily comprehend referenced circuitous impacts of accomplice support on post birth anxiety.

In synopsis, in spite of the fact that there have been a couple of clashing discoveries in the writing, countless examinations reliably indicated that accomplice support was related with post pregnancy anxiety and furthermore even may be one of the pre-birth hazard variables of post pregnancy anxiety. Lower levels of apparent accomplice support appear to expand the danger of creating burdensome indications in the baby blues period for ladies. Regardless of the requirement for more data on the instruments of impact, apparently deficient accomplice backing might be a hazard factor for sadness in the baby blues period.

# Grown-up Romantic Attachment Patterns

Connection hypothesis offers a profoundly helpful hypothetical system for analysts to comprehend the adjustment procedure of ladies in the time of change to parenthood. As indicated by connection hypothesis, the newborn child creates "interior working models" about oneself as well as other people dependent on the nature of the association with his/her essential guardian and these inside working models decide the conduct and mentalities of the baby during adulthood in cozy connections, particularly in distressing circumstances. When it comes to the romantic attachments, the women can help a lot of support from their partners and also ensure that the babies are getting male attention.

Analysts have recommended that sentimental accomplices likewise serve comparative capacities as guardians do in youth, for example, fulfilling the requirements for closeness, a protected base and a place of refuge and they have additionally suggested that sentimental accomplices have distinctive connection styles. Thus, a few analysts have inspected grown-up sentimental connection designs as a hazard factor for post birth anxiety, recommending that 'interior working models' are particularly actuated in testing periods, for example, change to parenthood. At the point when writing on grown-up connection designs is analyzed, it creates the impression that particularly the uneasiness measurement of connection assumes a significant job in the improvement of post birth anxiety. In a longitudinal report tending to the progress to parenthood as far as burdensome side effects of guardians, have analyzed the job of unreliable connection in the burdensome manifestations of new moms.

The analysts likewise took comparative measures from a benchmark group of wedded couples without youngsters to think about unseasoned parents and the couples without kids as far as the adjustments in connection designs after some time. As indicated by the outcomes, the impact of connection nervousness on the burdensome side effects was more noteworthy for new moms than ladies without kids. In light of this discovering, it very well may be said that progress to parenthood process is so unpleasant and testing that it can enact the connection designs in ladies and particularly on edge connection makes new moms inclined to experience the ill effects of burdensome indications. In addition, considerably after an extraordinary number of other hazard factors considered to affect post pregnancy anxiety (e.g., low conjugal fulfillment and absence of social help) were controlled, connection nervousness despite everything kept on foreseeing post pregnancy anxiety in new moms. In any case, more critically, this connection between connection nervousness and post birth anxiety was directed by the manner in which that spouses react to their wives' requirement for care and backing.

At the end of the day, the relationship between connection uneasiness and burdensome manifestations were more noteworthy for ladies whose spouses detailed indicating less consideration. This finding recommends that the help and care gave by spouses can diminish the negative outcomes of connection uneasiness somewhat in new moms. Additionally, Simpson and associates found that apparent accomplice bolster assumed an intervening job in the connection among pre-birth and postnatal burdensome manifestations for ladies with on edge connection style. All the more explicitly, tensely joined ladies who showed more significant levels of burdensome side effects before labor apparent less help from their accomplices experiencing significant change to parenthood, which at that point prompted more significant levels of burdensome indications after labor. No such finding was found for the shirking measurement of connection.

Ladies with higher shaky connection were less happy with their accomplices' help, which thusly expanded the chance of post pregnancy anxiety. These discoveries both propose that accomplice support shows up as a significant factor clarifying the connection between uncertain connection and post pregnancy anxiety and explain how two hazard factors tended to right now (i.e., shaky connection and accomplice support) affect post pregnancy anxiety together. In another examination, baby blues moms and non-postpartum moms were thought about as far as connection designs, confidence and burdensome manifestations. This investigation uncovered that confidence assumed a middle person job in the relationship between engrossed connection style and sadness seriousness; this relationship was watched distinctly in moms were in the baby blues period.

Baby blues moms with distracted connection style had lower levels of confidence, which thusly expanded the chance of having burdensome indications. Another finding was added to the writing which reveals insight into the potential systems in the connection between these factors. Also, in an examination directed by Lee and Koo (2015), the arbiter job of self-esteem in the connection between grown-up sentimental connection designs and post pregnancy anxiety was researched. In addition, the arbitrator job of moms' parental self-efficacy on the intervening impacts of confidence was additionally analyzed.

Results exhibited that confidence went about as a full go between in the connection between engrossed connection and post birth anxiety, while it went about as an incomplete middle person job in the connection between frightful connection and post pregnancy anxiety. Notwithstanding, more critically, the go between a job of confidence in the connections between shaky connections (engrossed and frightful) and post maternal self-adequacy directed birth anxiety. Considering these discoveries, it is reasoned that not all moms with a shaky connection style (engrossed or frightful) will show burdensome side effects through low confidence; rather, having a high parental self-viability shields moms from the danger of creating burdensome indications. A high impression of maternal self-adequacy has all the earmarks of being a defensive factor in the connection between shaky connection and post birth anxiety in which confidence went about as a middle person.

Then again, in an ongoing longitudinal examination, Clout and Brown (2016) researched the job of connection measurements and conjugal quality in baby blues pressure, uneasiness, and burdensome indications and gained clashing outcomes with the past discoveries in the writing. In the light of past research discoveries, scientists estimated that connection uneasiness in the last trimester of pregnancy would foresee burdensome indications at 4-6 months baby blues.

They arrived at the resolution that neither general-connection nor conjugal explicit connection designs did not expect post birth anxiety. When you are preparing for a baby, you need to make sure that you talk to the partner about their role and how they can help you during this time. Then again, as per intervention investigations, conjugal fulfillment went about as a full go between connection tension and post birth anxiety. In spite of the fact that the tension element of connection does not directly affect post birth anxiety, the low conjugal fulfillment has all the earmarks of being the instrument that gives the connection between connection nervousness and post birth anxiety. New moms with high connection nervousness were seen as inclined to post birth anxiety just when they experienced issues with conjugal connections. In another examination, the impacts of both current social troubles (low conjugal fulfillment and unreliable connection) and negative youth encounters on post birth anxiety were researched to comprehend the procedures that influence post birth anxiety from a more extensive point of view. We uncovered that on edge connection was a critical indicator of sadness at a year baby blues.

There is a connection between the baby blues and the mothers' unavailability to take care of her baby. In view of these discoveries, it very well may be said that on edge connection assumes a fundamental job in the upkeep of post birth anxiety. In a later report, the go between the job of post pregnancy anxiety in the connection between new moms' grown-up sentimental connection styles and mother-newborn child connection challenges was researched. The outcomes yielded that post birth anxiety intervened the connection between just the restless/undecided connection style and newborn child centered nervousness. This finding was reliable with past discoveries proposing that connection tension was an increasingly compelling variable on post birth anxiety when contrasted with connection evasion. The notable steady connection between unreliable connection designs and post birth anxiety in Western nations has been researched in non-western societies too as of late.

In an examination led in Japan, steady with past research discoveries, we discovered that uncertain connection designs were a critical indicator of post birth anxiety. Besides, an examination directed in Turkey additionally upheld the positive connection between shaky connection designs and post birth anxiety manifestations. In rundown, an extraordinary number of concentrates upheld that particularly the tension component of connection assumes a significant job in the improvement of post birth anxiety. While a few examinations research just the immediate impact of connection tension on post pregnancy anxiety, the potential instruments that may underlie the connection between these two factors have caught the consideration of certain scientists.

Accomplice support is one of these components that represents this relationship. Since people with high connection nervousness don't see themselves as deserving of being adored and give outrageous significance to cozy connections, they may feel as though their relationship is tried by a significant life stressor, for example, change to parenthood. On the off chance that they feel that they don't get the normal consideration and backing from their life partners, this procedure can be progressively distressing. These people may be progressively inclined to create post birth anxiety. These discoveries bolster the perspective on Bowlby (1988), the pioneer of connection hypothesis, proposing that restlessly joined ladies who figure they don't get the normal help from their spouses during the progress to parenthood are bound to create post birth anxiety.

Notwithstanding saw accomplice support, confidence, conjugal fulfillment, and impression of parental self-viability are among the components that underlie the connection between connection uneasiness and post pregnancy anxiety. These exploration discoveries bolster that the connection between unreliable connection and post pregnancy anxiety has in certainty a perplexing nature and it is critical to research the potential systems that underlie this connection.

# Conclusion:

By now you know that postpartum disorders can affect anyone. It's true that there are some predictors that can help the doctors to screen pregnant women in a better way but this ailment can affect women of all backgrounds. No matter if you are rich, poor, have a happy family, or are a single parent, postpartum can affect you in a number of ways.

After reading this book, you can easily differentiate postpartum depression from baby blues and make necessary steps to live a happy life. We have also discussed the role of a partner during postpartum. This book is not only geared towards the new mothers but also provide insight on how the doctors and partners can help the new mothers in getting their life back on track after childbirth.

Because of PPD, most women feel empty and alone. You need to be prepared to face this time as this is temporary and by following the tips mentioned in the book, you can easily bring your life back on track.

Reviews are not easy to come by.

As an independent staff with a tiny marketing budget, we rely on readers, like you, to leave a short review on Amazon.

Even if it's just a sentence or two!

**Customer Reviews**

★★★★★ 2
5.0 out of 5 stars ▼

| | | |
|---|---|---|
| 5 star | ▬▬▬▬▬ | 100% |
| 4 star | | 0% |
| 3 star | | 0% |
| 2 star | | 0% |
| 1 star | | 0% |

Share your thoughts with other customers

[ Write a customer review ]  ⬅

See all verified purchase reviews ›

So if you enjoyed the book, please...

>> Click here to leave a brief review on Amazon.

We are very appreciative for your review as it truly makes a difference.

Thank you from the bottom of our hearts for purchasing this book and reading it to the end.

**THANK YOU FOR PURCHASING THIS AMAZING MASTERPIECE FOR PREGNANT WOMEN AND FIRST-TIME MOMS IN THE MOMMY'S ANGELS BOOK COLLECTIONS**

**MOMMY'S ANGELS Book Series** was inspired to take the guesswork out of motherhood and childcare. In most cases, from the moment a couple finds out that they are pregnant, their greatest desire is to gather all possible information about pregnancy and motherhood – to avoid being caught up by surprise. As it is often far much better to know what possible problems you may be confronted with, and be prepared and to solve them; as compared to being in the dark.

**MOMMY'S ANGELS Book Collections** offer some of the most reliable pieces of information that are dedicated to motherhood, many of which have been the true saviors and sure guide for first-time parents. We have received lots of pleasant feedbacks from mothers and, even, fathers who were able to stay calmer reading a book that walks them through each phase of their parenting journey.

You will also find titles that are dedicated to the modern mother who wants to take care of her pregnancy and motherhood, without neglecting her style and femininity.

Like other **MOMMY'S ANGELS Book Series,** the comments, stories, and experiences of pediatricians, psychologists, gynecologists and other mothers like you, contained in this book will help you enjoy the best adventure of your life.

I look forward to hearing your testimonies and awesome feedbacks. **Cheers!!**

## MOMMY'S ANGELS
EDITORIAL STAFF
GROW YOUR TODDLER TO THE BEST!